Yoga fun

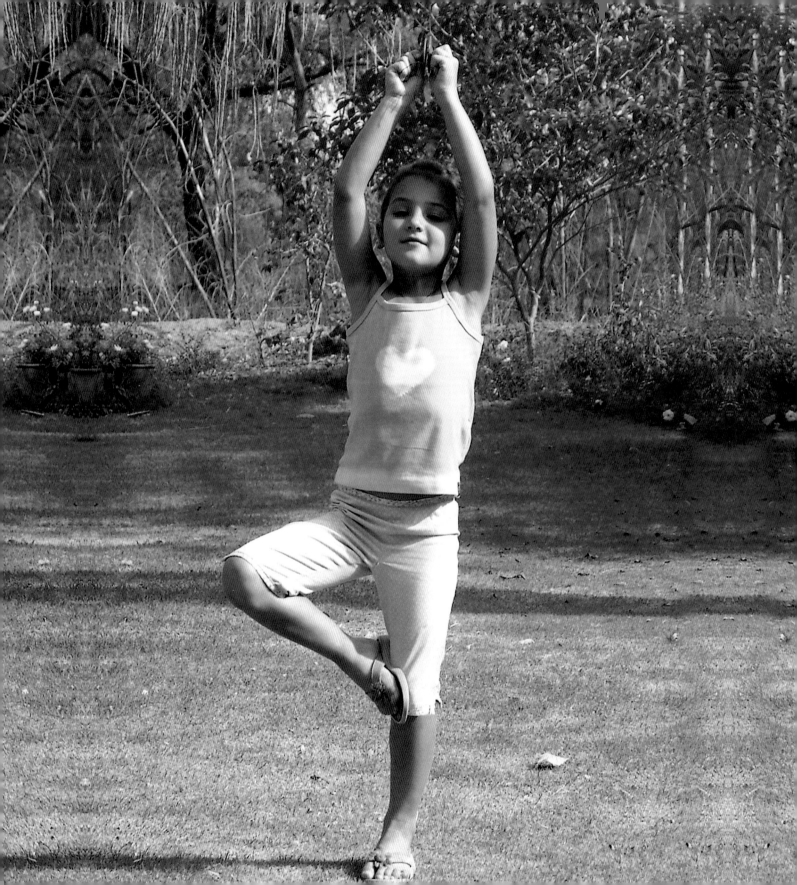

Yoga fun
for toddlers, children, & you

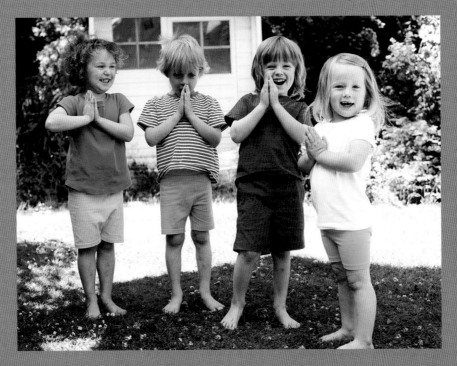

JULIET PEGRUM

CICO BOOKS
LONDON NEW YORK

Published in 2010 by CICO Books
an imprint of Ryland Peters & Small
20–21 Jockey's Fields   519 Broadway, 5th Floor
London WC1R 4BW   New York NY 10012

10 9 8 7 6 5 4 3 2 1

A CIP catalog record for this book is available from the Library of Congress and the British Library.

ISBN-13: 978-1-907030-14-7

A previous edition of this book was published under the title Children's Yoga (ISBN-13: 978-1-903116-95-1).

Printed in China

Project editor: Mary Lambert
Designer: Barbara Zuñiga
Photographer: Ian Boddy, pages 3, 5, 7, 11, 12, 20, 23, 25, 30, 33, 42, 51 (left and right), 60, 80, 96, 102, 105 (below), 110, 116; all other images by Sandra Lousada

AUTHOR'S ACKNOWLEDGMENTS

I would like to thank Bel Gibbs for her help in finding child models. I would also personally like to thank: Hal, Brogan, Nicholas, Oliver, Georgia, Brittany, Ambessa, Ayana, Alicia, Darragh, Gabriella, Joe, Timmy, Robert, William, Max, Alex, Lydia, Rosie, Tao tao, Imogen and Sophie for their tireless energy and enthusiasm in demonstrating the poses for this book. I would also like to thank Mary Lambert for skillfully organizing the material, and Sandra Lousada for her wonderful photographs.

Juliet Pegrum can be contacted at:
julietpegrum@mahamudrayoga.com

With many thanks to the following additional models: Jude, Clarissa, Xanthe, Amelia, Cece, and Felix.

Contents

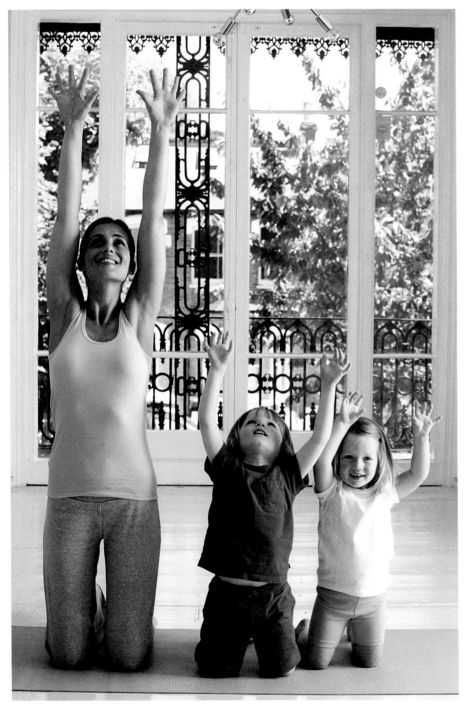

Introduction

Yoga is a timeless and practical technique for developing both the mind and body. The poses in this book are particularly good for energetic children as they will enjoy the physical exertion, and will also benefit from the body and mind development. The different postures are specially adapted so that young children can also enjoy practicing yoga.

This chapter shows how practicing yoga regularly can help a child develop better body and mind awareness and breathing habits, and discusses how yoga improves and balances the functioning of the body's glandular system and the chakras—the body's spiritual energy centers.

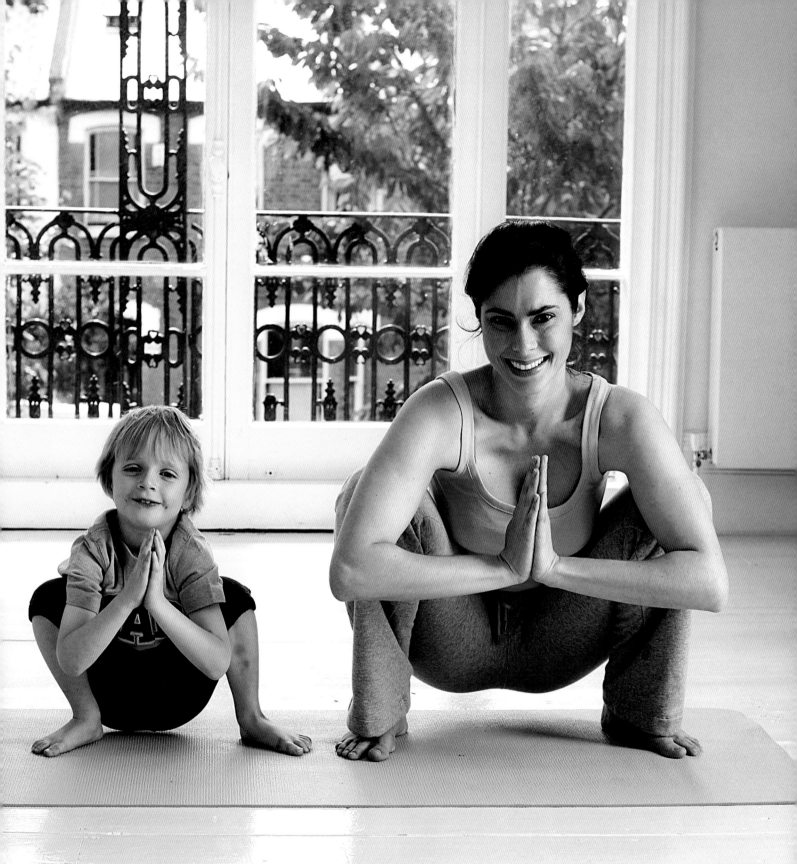

Yoga and children

The yoga system was devised in India thousands of years ago. Yoga *asanas*, or poses, are derived from observing nature. The yogis studied the movements of animals, noting how they breathed, moved, and relaxed. Many of the yoga poses imitate or represent the spirit of animals, such as the dog, lion, or cat. They also imitate parts of the environment, such as mountains or trees, helping us to appreciate the grace of these natural wonders. Performing the animal poses in yoga shows us that to reach our highest potential as human beings and show loving, compassionate, forgiving, and happy characteristics, we need to control our baser animal instincts, such as greed, selfishness and desire.

Hatha yoga poses

Included in this book are simple hatha yoga practices that incorporate: physical poses, breathing techniques, chanting, and concentration exercises. Movement is essential for growing bodies, as it is the only activity that connects the two hemispheres of the brain and helps the brain to develop to its full potential. As a parent, use the information in this book to practice the poses at home with your children. Different workouts are included on pages 116–127. Poses that are good for young children and beginners are also indicated. Putting 20 minutes aside, two or three times a week, to practice yoga with your children is a great way to nurture them and spend valuable time together as a family. Yoga also helps mothers to stay in shape, so it is a good excuse for you to practice regularly with your children. It is a good idea to take a few classes locally first so that you can share the poses confidently with your children. As the children improve and perform the yoga poses more confidently, they too may want to attend a local class so that they can interact with other children and also advance further with their yoga technique.

How yoga helps children

When children practice yoga it can help them get in touch with nature and the normal rhythms of life. It can encourage them to become gentle and kind adults, who will hopefully create a more peaceful world in the future. When older children practice yoga, it helps to keep their bones healthy and strong and their muscles supple and flexible, aiding their physical performance in sports. The balancing poses can increase their mental focus and concentration and awaken their creativity. Regularly doing the poses can also control and soothe their emotions, letting them rest more easily and sleep soundly. It can also preserve their youthfulness: yogis in India who have practiced yoga all their lives have a young and ageless appearance. Most children love to practice yoga, as many of the postures imitate nature and animals, plus it is also a fun, non-competitive activity. Try to establish a healthy, regular, and enjoyable yoga routine with your children from a young age, as it is much harder to impose set routines as they get older.

Traditionally in India, a proper yoga routine is introduced to a child in his eighth year, as this is seen as the beginning of puberty, starting him on the path toward adulthood. Also, at this age the air sacs, or alveoli, in the lungs are fully developed for the breathing exercises, and the child has gained the ability to conceptualize.

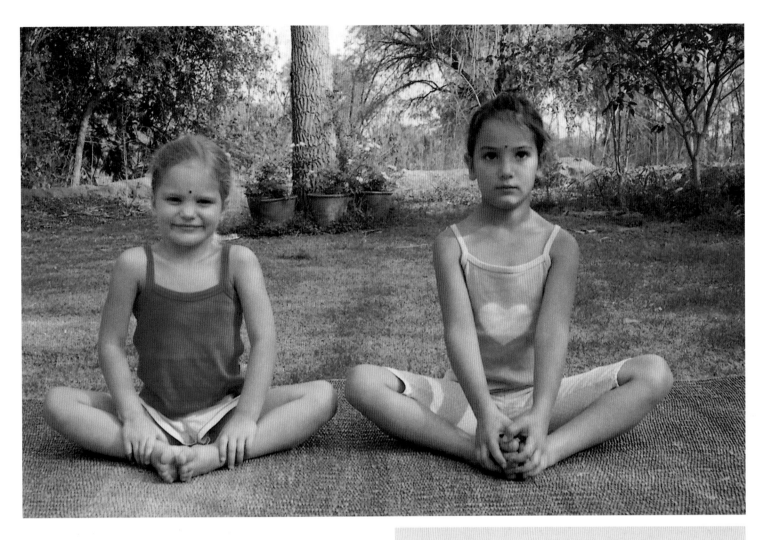

Learning yoga from a young age can help a child become more supple and mentally focused.

Yoga for younger children

Yoga can also be taught to children who are three to six years old, but it is best to give the poses and practices a fun element so that it stimulates their creative thinking and intellectual growth. So yoga for this young age group is most effective through guided play, which may involve their senses. You can also use inventive games that capture their imagination and focuses their attention. Using playful techniques with children is a powerful form of teaching that has been used by many different cultures for centuries.

SAFETY BOX

- Always be present to practice yoga with your child or children in a warm, open space, clear of any sharp objects, furniture, or breakable items.

- Make sure that your child breathes steadily during each pose and does not try to hold her breath.

- If any pose is painful or uncomfortable, do not let your child overstretch; let him build up his flexibility over time.

- Remind your child to lengthen and elongate her spine during the poses.

- Always practice yoga together at least two hours after a meal.

Benefits of yoga for children

Yoga is a wonderful movement discipline that can give your children regular exercise. It can also keep them toned and supple, with joints that work to their full range of motion. This is especially important today, as children are spending more time than ever in sedentary activities such as watching TV, listening to music or playing computer games. Research shows that the long-term effects of a sedentary lifestyle are clearly linked to high blood pressure, obesity, ulcers, and poor functioning of the heart and lungs.

Yoga takes a holistic approach to maintaining health and wellbeing that makes your children feel good and aids their growing bodies. Studies into the benefits of yoga have shown that it can help children in the following ways.

Flexibility and strength

Children are naturally flexible and agile, and these are important qualities to maintain in their young bodies. Yoga poses, or *asanas*, strengthen their growing spines, keep their muscles supple, and encourage good joint movement. The action of the poses creates a more elaborate range of muscle motor skills that fine-tune coordination and increase the overall range of motion.

On a deeper level, the intense bending and twisting movements in the poses stimulate and massage the internal organs, balancing the endocrine and other bodily systems. Certain poses stimulate different areas of the body: for example, Candle pose (shoulder stand, see page 75) helps the functioning of the thyroid and parathyroid glands.

Yoga poses combine well with sports, as they help flexible children to become stronger and build endurance. They also help less supple children who do a lot of sports to gain greater flexibility. Many training and stretching exercises are, in fact, borrowed from yoga.

Better posture

Practicing the poses regularly straightens and strengthens the spine, sending a fresh flow of blood and nutrients to a child's muscles and disks. When the back is upright and lifted, it enables better energy flow, and the nervous system works more efficiently, improving such involuntary actions as breathing or digestion. Performing the yoga poses also improves and strengthens the muscles that support the spine, reducing the likelihood of backache. Even a slight improvement in posture greatly enhances lung capacity, blood circulation, and energy flow through the body.

If children develop good posture from practicing yoga, it can counteract the time they spend slumped in a chair watching TV or using a computer. Regularly sitting in a slouched posture also prevents children from breathing properly.

Body awareness

Yoga encourages body awareness through the poses, as most of them are repeated on both sides of the body, which is believed to harmonize the left and right hemispheres of the brain. The ability to distinguish between left and right is the essence of body awareness that develops around the age of seven, about the time that hand dominance is established.

Performing dynamic sequences such as the Warrior on pages 88–89 strengthens the legs, hips, and back.

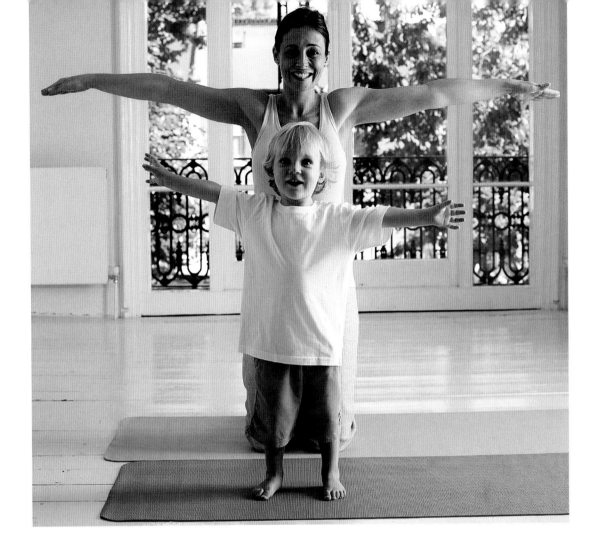

Breathing

Learning how to breathe properly is an essential part of yoga practice that is explained fully on pages 102–109.

Breathing is one of our most important functions in life. Babies naturally breathe deeply from their diaphragms, but as we get older and have more stress in our lives, we tend to breathe more shallowly from our chests. Teaching children to breathe more deeply in yoga allows the body to draw in more *prana*: the subtle, life-sustaining energy that is taken into the body thro ugh air, sunshine, water and food.

Breathing has a direct link with our mind and emotions. When we feel nervous or upset, our breathing becomes very shallow and labored. Practicing breathing deeply helps to calm the mind and frees any blocked emotions or creative energy.

Yoga breathing techniques can encourage better sleeping patterns. Letting a child practice the Relaxed tummy breath exercise (see page 105) before bed can disperse a buildup of nervous energy so that he or she can completely relax.

Concentration techniques

Focusing the mind is an essential part of yoga practice that is described in more detail in Chapter 8 (see pages 110–115). Concentration and visualization exercises help children to learn to sit still, get in touch with their inner selves, focus their minds and avoid outside distractions so that they enjoy the present moment. When they acquire concentration skills, they are more alert and receptive, making it easier for them to pay attention at school and increase their learning abilities.

The brain is split into two cerebral hemispheres, with each side having a unique function. The yoga poses, the breathing exercises, and the concentration techniques also help to balance and stimulate both hemispheres of the brain: the left, logical, and rational side and the right, more imaginative, creative, and intuitive side.

Communication skills

Children's speech development relates to their intellectual abilities, so some will learn to speak earlier than others. They are stimulated to speak by the "conversations" they have with their parents and other children. Their speech is then further developed by teachers and by learning from the world around them. Yoga can develop children's vocabulary, as it teaches them the names of animals, parts of the body, and objects as they practice all the poses. Chanting or singing can be fun and enjoyable to do, and they also develop communication skills.

Practicing simple yoga poses from an early age can help to develop a child's confidence and self-esteem.

Building self-esteem

When you have a positive self-image you radiate self-confidence and joy. Studies into the use of positive affirmations (saying a positive phrase repeatedly) have shown that your personality reflects how you see yourself. If a child feels inadequate, he or she will act according to this self-image. Yoga uses positive language, affirmations, and visualization techniques that increase a child's self-esteem. In addition, as a child becomes more proficient at the yoga poses, he feels more healthy and toned and his confidence and self-image improve.

A non-competitive discipline

Yoga is non-competitive, so children can enjoy the physical and mental exercises without worrying about succeeding or failing. Playing competitive sports can make some children stressed and anxious. When teaching yoga poses, do not use negative language, such as "That's wrong," or demand perfection. It is far better to instill a joy of practicing the techniques.

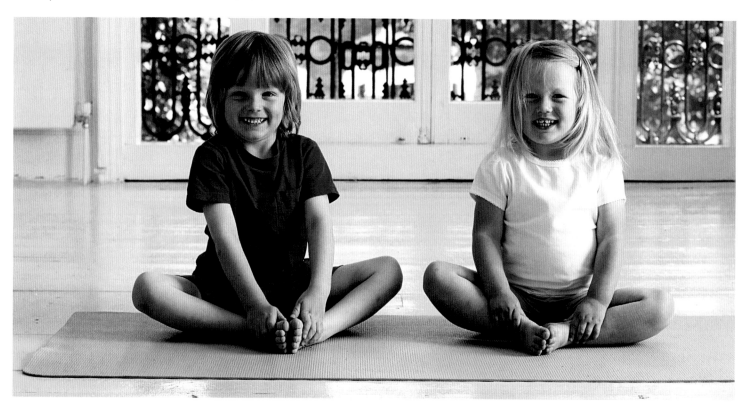

YOGA PHILOSOPHY

In yoga philosophy, there are suggested guidelines for how to live. There are five actions that we should avoid, called *yamas*, and five actions to adopt, called *niyamas*. These actions are important for children to learn, as they are an integral part of yoga practice. They also teach us to act responsibly and to make the most of ourselves.

Step 1 Yamas
RESTRAINTS

Ahimsa—not being violent is an attitude of not wanting to harm any living being, including yourself, in word, thought, or action. It is important to teach children to be kind, to others and to themselves.

Satya—not trying to be what you are not, it is about leading an honest and open life.

Asteya—literally meaning "to not steal," this *yama* is about not being jealous of others or taking or using anything that is not freely given.

Brahmacarya—conservation of energy; controlling the senses so that you avoid overindulgences, such as eating too much.

Aparigraha—avoiding being greedy or hoarding, or hankering after the possessions of others.

Step 2 Niyamas
OBSERVANCES

Saucha—staying clean: inside your body and your home.

Santosha—contentment: being happy as you are, and with what you have.

Tapas—self-discipline: making the most of yourself, pursuing worthwhile goals, and not giving up too easily.

Svadhyaya—worthwhile study and learning.

Ishvarapranidhana—surrender: dedicating all you do and achieve to others.

Yoga ethics

Yoga is not a religion, but a way of life—although it does have some basic ethics used by many religions. The main principle of yoga is: "Do unto others as you would have others do unto you," so not harming other living creatures, physically, verbally or mentally, is the basic principle of yoga.

Children learn moral judgment by responding to older children and adults who act as role models. When children learn yoga, it teaches them to respect themselves and other children. It helps them understand how their actions impact on others, and it also lets them appreciate the wonders of the natural world.

Yoga for your mind, body, and spirit

Our bodies are complex systems that comprise numerous working parts, such as the arms, legs, heart, the respiratory, circulatory, and digestive systems. When any part of the body is not functioning properly, it affects us both physically and spiritually.

Western medicine focuses on treating physical symptoms, whereas in eastern medicine and in the yoga system, the body is viewed energetically. *Prana* is a subtle vital force or energy that is everywhere. Our bodies take in *prana* from the world around us, from the food that we eat, the air that we breathe, and from sunlight. This energy then flows through all the major organs and body parts via the chakras (our spiritual energy centers) and energy channels called *nadis*—there are 72,000 in all. The word *nadi* literally means flow, and to be healthy, energy must flow freely along these channels to the body organs, glands, and spiritual centers. Yoga is a profound system of exercise that stimulates the body physically, mentally, and energetically.

The endocrine system

One of the unique qualities of yoga is how it affects the endocrine system. The endocrine system, or glandular system, controls the body's functions, secreting hormones directly into the bloodstream. The hormones are chemical messengers, giving commands from the brain to the body. They not only affect how well the body functions, but also influence our moods and behavior, sometimes making us feeling angry, depressed, happy, or sad.

Growth in children

How well the endocrine system is working is particularly important in children, as it determines how fast they grow and their emotional health. Also, around the age of eight, the controlling pineal gland slows down and the pituitary takes over, sending reproductive hormones into the body that set off a rapid growth in emotional and mental capabilities. These hormones then eventually stimulate the onset of puberty. When a child practices yoga regularly, the endocrine system is kept in balance, and she grows and develops normally. But if there is a blockage in the hormonal system, such as an under- or overactive thyroid, a child can change and become either sluggish or hyperactive.

Yoga poses also increase the intake of oxygen into the bloodstream, boosting the blood flow to the glandular areas, making them function more efficiently and improving overall health and wellbeing.

The poses can be performed to either slow down or energize the system. If a child suffers from hyperactivity, you can introduce calm breathing exercises or relaxation techniques (see Chapters 7 and 8). Hyperactive children, or children suffering from attention-deficit disorder, can often become balanced naturally through doing yoga. A child who seems dull and listless can boost her bodily functions by doing some dynamic or energetic poses.

When yoga is practiced during puberty, it can help to regulate the physical changes and the hormonal surges that are taking place in the body. This regulation of the body can in turn reduce the unpredictable mood swings that seem to affect many teenagers.

The endocrine glands

There are eight different kinds of glands in the body, each with a different function.

Pituitary gland This is located in the head. It is the master gland of the body, as all information feeds back to the pituitary gland and it controls all the other glands. It influences overall body growth, and how the other glands and organs function.

Pineal gland This is also situated in the head. Little is known about the pineal gland, which is located in the *Medulla oblongata* (the lowest part of the brainstem). It is active in the development of children until the age of eight, when it begins to calcify. As it becomes less active, the pituitary gland begins to take over, marking the start of puberty.

Thyroid and parathyroid glands These glands are located in the throat. The thyroid is responsible for physical and mental growth, heart rate, metabolism, blood pressure, and glucose absorption. The secretions of the parathyroid gland control the calcium levels in the blood that affect bone strength, muscle tone, and the nervous system.

Thymus gland This is located in the heart region. It is active during a child's formative years, stimulating immune-system response and encouraging normal body growth. It starts to shrink and diminish at puberty, around the age of 14.

Adrenal glands These are situated above the kidneys, and release hormones in the system such as hydrocortisone to regulate the metabolism, and adrenaline to trigger the body's response to stress: the fight or flight mechanism.

Testes and ovaries These are the sexual glands of the body. The male testes and female ovaries govern the smooth functioning of the reproductive organs. The testes control the growth of body hair, body size, and the tone of voice. Estrogen is a female hormone produced by the ovaries. Estrogen plays important roles in puberty—controlling the menstrual cycle—and in reproduction and maintaining healthy bones.

In the same way that a well-maintained car operates, the smooth functioning of the endocrine glands ensures that the body "runs" well.

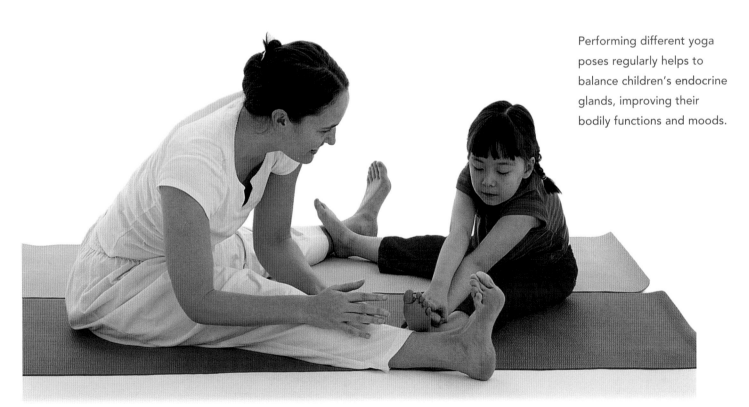

Performing different yoga poses regularly helps to balance children's endocrine glands, improving their bodily functions and moods.

THE ETHERIC BODY

The Chakras

The endocrine glands are intrinsically linked to the chakras (our spiritual energy centers). So if a chakra malfunctions, there will also be hormonal, physical, and emotional disturbance. The word chakra literally means "wheel" or "disk," as the chakras are tight circles of energy. Seven major chakras are located in the aura (the etheric body) along the spinal column from the base of the spine to the crown of the head. In the yoga system, each chakra links to emotional, psychological, and spiritual development. All the chakras are joined together by *nadis* (energy channels). How each chakra functions depends on the person's spiritual and physical health, so some may be underactive, sluggish, or possibly hyperactive. Practicing yoga can help to shift energetic blockages and bring the chakras back in balance.

Balancing CHILDREN'S chakras

Performing the yoga poses and doing the breathing exercises (see Chapter 7) can purify children's chakras and help to harmonize *prana*, allowing it to move freely through the body. This allows them to develop physically, emotionally, and psychologically, so that they reach their highest potential.

The seven chakras

1 *MULADHARA* (ROOT) CHAKRA

This is the lowest chakra, situated in the lower pelvic floor, between the anus and sexual organs. In yoga, *Muladhara* is shown as a beautiful red lotus with four petals. In the center of the lotus is a yellow square that represents the Earth element and *shakti*, or primal energy.

Physically, it is believed in yoga to be connected to a gland that no longer exists, while emotionally it is about basic human survival, feeling stable and safe in this world. When this chakra is functioning properly, a child feels grounded, is full of energy, and gets on well with other children and adults. If it is overactive, she can become very selfish or self-centered, be a bully to other children, or be too boisterous; if it is underactive, she may be needy, fearful, and suffer from low selfesteem or a bad self-image.

To balance the *Muladhara* chakra, practice Bridge pose (see page 71) and Locust pose (see page 56).

2 *SVADHISTHANA* (SACRAL) CHAKRA

The second chakra is located in the pelvis, just above the first, around the area of the prostate gland or uterus. *Svadhisthana* literally means "an abode of one's own." It is represented by an orange lotus with six petals. At the center of the lotus is a silver crescent moon, denoting the Water element.

Physically, it relates to the ovaries or testes, while emotionally it is about the need to find your identity. It can be about the attraction

The Chakras

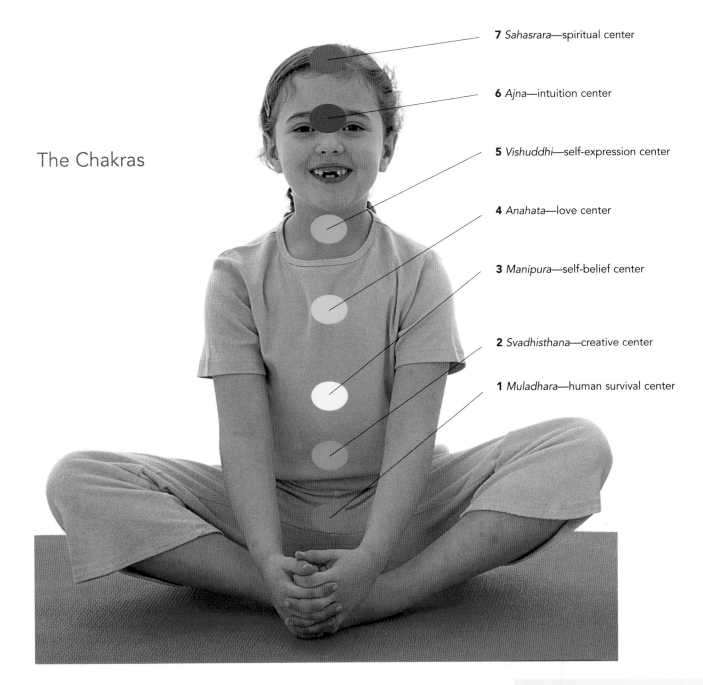

7 *Sahasrara*—spiritual center

6 *Ajna*—intuition center

5 *Vishuddhi*—self-expression center

4 *Anahata*—love center

3 *Manipura*—self-belief center

2 *Svadhisthana*—creative center

1 *Muladhara*—human survival center

of opposites, how you relate to friends, family, and partners. It is your creative center and represents fertility. When this chakra is balanced, a child is completely in tune with her feelings, is imaginative, and trusts the actions of other people. If it is overactive, she can become too emotional and be manipulative; if it is underactive, she can be bored, disinterested, and self-critical.

To balance the *Svadisthana* chakra, practice Butterfly pose (see page 57), Knee to chest warm-up (see page 38), and Chair pose (see page 67).

3 MANIPURA (SOLAR PLEXUS) CHAKRA

This is the third chakra, situated in the upper abdomen behind the navel, or Solar Plexus area. It is the center of heat and vitality, the area of the body where food is transformed into energy. *Manipura* literally means "lustrous gem" or "city of jewels." It is depicted as a bright yellow lotus with ten petals. Within the lotus is a red triangle, representing the Fire element.

Physically, it is associated with the pancreas, while emotionally it deals with our will power and self-belief: how we use our basic creative energies. When this chakra is balanced, a child respects himself and other people, is energetic, spontaneous, and loves seeing friends. If it is overactive, he may be angry, controlling, or just ill tempered and dominating; if it is underactive, he can be frightened, insecure, painfully shy, and need constant reassurance.

To balance the *Manipura* chakra, practice Row the boat pose (see page 90), Bicycle pose (see page 91), and Boat pose (see page 68).

4 ANAHATA (HEART) CHAKRA

This chakra is in the center of the chest, near the heart. *Anahata* literally means "unstruck sound" and refers to the life beat of the Universe, similar to the body's heartbeat: the pulse of life and love. This love is unconditional, constant, and pure. The chakra is shown as a blue lotus with 12 petals. In the center of the lotus are two interlocking triangles representing the Air element.

Physically, it links to the thymus, while emotionally it holds our powerful emotions, such as love, compassion, patience, and contentment. When it is functioning well, a child is caring and nurturing, can show compassion to others, and is contented. If it is overactive, she can become possessive, be divisive, or act melodramatically; If it is underactive, she may be spiteful, shut down emotionally, or have a fear of being rejected.

To balance the *Anahata* chakra, practice Bridge pose (see page 71), Bow pose (see page 72), Cobra pose (see page 53), and Wheel pose (see page 73).

5 VISHUDDHI (THROAT) CHAKRA

This chakra is located in the throat, close to the larynx. *Vishuddhi* means "purification through words," such as by reciting a mantra. It is represented by a violet lotus containing 16 petals. In the center of the lotus is a large white circle that represents the element of Ether, or Space. The throat chakra links to self-expression, and is said to be the bridge that exists between the body and the head.

Physically, it corresponds to the thyroid and parathyroids, while emotionally it is the communication center, giving us the ability to speak the truth and express all our ideas creatively. The lesson of the fifth chakra is to be able to take responsibility for yourself and your actions. When the throat chakra is balanced, a child will communicate well, be able to express herself verbally, and be willing to listen attentively to others. If it is overactive, she may be a chatterbox, or a show-off who is always talking and who has a tendency to exaggerate events; if it is underactive, she may not say much or participate well in group activities.

To balance the *Vishuddhi* chakra, practice Candle pose (see page 75), Plow pose (see page 77), and Fish pose (see page 59).

6 AJNA (THIRD EYE) CHAKRA

The *Ajna* chakra is in the middle of the forehead. *Ajna* means "to know," and is associated with your sixth sense or intuition. It is shown as a silver lotus with two petals. The two petals represent the two hemispheres of the brain that are portrayed as male and female energies: one being receptive, the other being dynamic.

Physically, it is associated with the pituitary and pineal glands, while emotionally it links to intuition, intelligence, concentration and visualization. When it is functioning well, a child will easily grasp concepts, be mentally alert, and have a charismatic personality that allows him to make friends easily. If it is overactive, he will be inattentive and unable to concentrate on anything; if it is underactive, she may have little personality or suffer from some learning problems or disabilities.

To improve the *Ajna* chakra, practice Upside-down tree pose (see page 74), Balancing stick pose (see page 65), and the visualization and concentration exercises (see Chapter 8).

7 SAHASRARA (CROWN) CHAKRA

This chakra is located on the crown of the head. It connects us to our spiritual side and our higher wisdom. It is shown as a lotus with a thousand petals, in the center of which is a *shivalingham*—a symbol of pure consciousness.

Physically, the *Sahasrara* chakra is connected to the pineal gland, while emotionally it connects to purity and spirit. When this chakra is balanced, a child will be at peace with herself and have a magnetic personality. If it is overactive, a child can act manically; if it is underactive, she may feel isolated or fear any sort of change.

To balance the *Sahasrara* chakra, practice the Concentration and visualization exercises (see Chapter 8). Meditation is also a good discipline to learn, as the child gets older.

The Aura

According to the Eastern system, the aura consists of five etheric layers or sheaths. Performing yoga can reconnect and harmonize these different bodies.

The first layer, or body, is called the food body or physical body. The food we eat affects the physical body; so if we have overeaten, the body becomes tired and lethargic and we can find it hard to concentrate. Also, if we do not exercise regularly and take care of our physical bodies, we can create imbalance. The yoga postures show children how they can tone and strengthen their physical bodies to stay fit and supple.

The second layer is the breath body or energetic body. Our brains require more oxygen than any other organ in the body to function well. When we breathe shallowly from our chests, or if there is a blockage, it affects the functioning of our mental and physical abilities. Yoga breathing exercises teach children the best way to breathe and how to stay healthy by breathing deeply from the diaphragm.

The third layer is the mental body, which comprises the conscious, subconscious, and instinctive parts of the mind. If your mind is unfocused and distracted, it makes it impossible to concentrate, and it also affects your breathing so that the physical body suffers. If children practice the Concentration exercises (see Chapter 8), they learn how to focus their minds, control their wellbeing, and study well at school and achieve their goals.

The fourth layer is the wisdom body, which relates to our intuition and higher understanding. The wisdom body is also connected to our emotions. So, if we are upset or depressed we may lack any inner drive or motivation. The yoga teachings and chanting practices can help children learn how to develop inner growth, balance their emotions, and keep them under control.

The fifth body is called the bliss body and is the subtlest layer. When all the other bodies are harmonized, the fifth body gives out joy, happiness, unconditional love, and fulfillment—the ideal state for all, particularly a child.

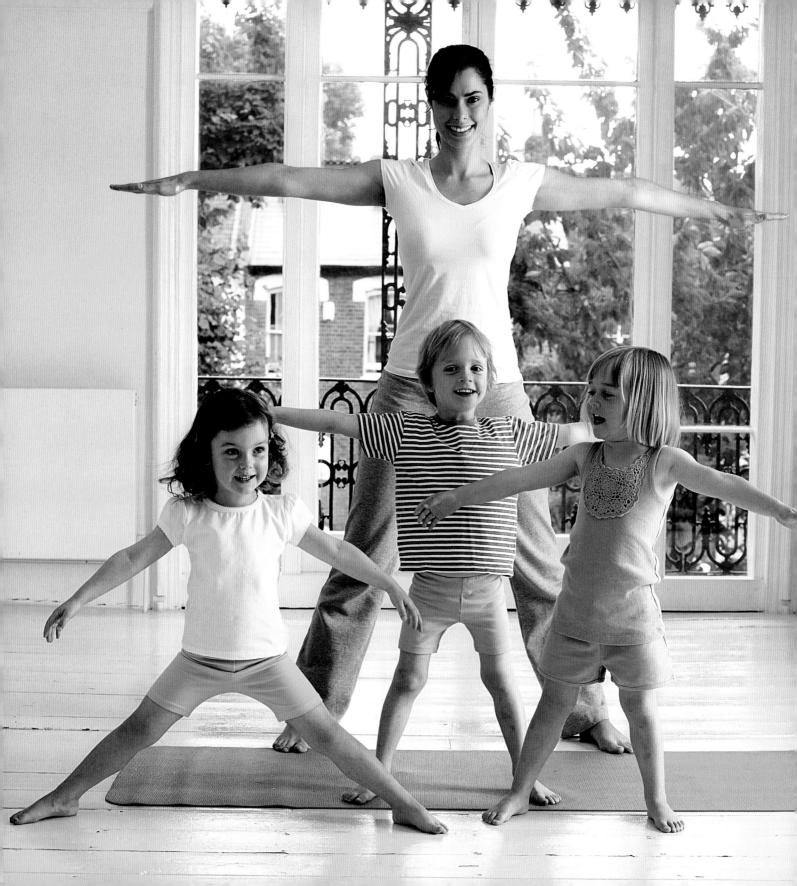

Chapter 1
Working with Kids

When you practice yoga with your children, you need to work with them as two different age groups: young children aged 3–6 and older children aged 7–11. With the younger age group, you can show them some fun yoga poses to strengthen their developing muscles and bone structures. The older age group are more developed physically, so together you can attempt more dynamic yoga poses.

This chapter shows how you can use yoga with both young and older children, what equipment and space you need to get started, and how you can practice together safely.

Yoga for young children 3–6

The age of three is an important milestone in the development of a child. It marks the transition from a toddler to a young child. Between the ages of 3 and 6 a child's movements become smoother and more coordinated, which is why this is a good age for you as a parent to introduce basic yoga movements to develop her range of motion. Movement is essential to enable children's development. Researchers have found that it connects all the brain functions, and opens the channels of communication between the left and right hemispheres, which in turn helps the brain to grow normally.

Between the ages of 3 and 6 young children become more adventurous and begin to feel comfortable with new people and places. They start to cooperate with each other, so working in groups with other children at this stage is very important. Organizing informal yoga sessions at home can be a fun group activity for your pre-school kids, and can strengthen their developing muscles and bone structures. The session can also help their vocabulary, so make up some yoga stories, and help them to learn the names of animals (see Chapter 3).

Children at this young age have an attention span of about 8–10 minutes, so let them have a short break every ten minutes. They can only understand basic two-step directions, such as "raise your arms and wiggle your fingers," so keep all your instructions short and succinct. Perfecting the poses is not important for young children; it is far better that they explore and expand their range of movement in the spirit of yoga play. Building play into the yoga movements is an effective teaching method that works well for very young children. As they get bored easily, always keep the sessions short and varied—about 20 minutes is enough—and make sure they do not hold the poses too long.

Keep them safe

When practicing yoga with small children, it is especially important to make sure there are no sharp objects around, or furniture to bump against, so check out the room you are using first. Let them use a yoga mat or a rug to soften any falls.

Developing bodies

In this young age group, the nervous system is still developing, so you may find the children often burst into spurts of chaotic movement, which is fine; do not try to control it or expect them to follow the poses perfectly—let them have some fun. Young children can enjoy repeating a pose, so there is no need to limit how many times they practice it; constant repetition is how they learn.

Early development

During the first few years of life, tremendous physical and mental development is taking place. To capture young children's imaginations, make the yoga session a complete learning experience. Let them use their senses: bring in music, simple chanting, or singing, and let them use percussion instruments (see Chapter 8). You do not have to use traditional yoga chants in Sanskrit; make up some fun ones yourself.

Teach them to chant vowels or to repeat simple nursery rhymes. Be inventive—think up simple stories or use their favorite books to incorporate the different animal or object poses (see Chapters 3 and 4) that are shown in this book. Using these techniques will also help the children to develop their vocabulary, as by repeating the poses, they will remember the animals they are imitating.

Yoga games

Play a game such as musical statues, but when the music stops, get the children to adopt a yoga pose. Alternatively, pretend that you or one of the children is a wizard such as the book character Harry Potter, who can change them into different objects with the wave of his wand.

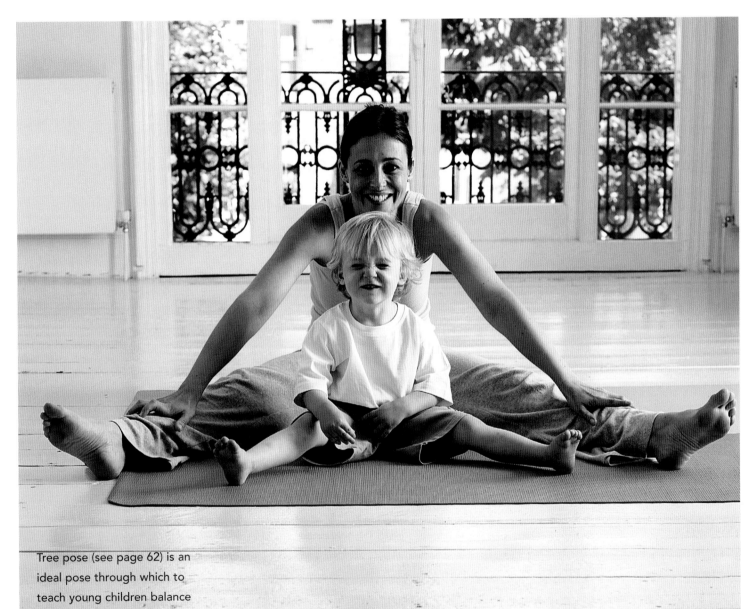

Tree pose (see page 62) is an ideal pose through which to teach young children balance and coordination.

Yoga for children 7–11

In India, yoga was seriously introduced to both boys and girls at the age of eight years. This was seen as the age when puberty began and they were starting their journeys toward adulthood. In the West from this age, yoga lessons can become more structured.

More formal yoga

Dynamic *asanas*, in which a series of different poses mixed together, such as Salute to the sun (see pages 82–84) and Warrior pose (see pages 88–89), can be taught to older children, along with more complex poses. By the time a child is eight, the air sacs or alveoli in the lungs are completely formed, although the lungs will continue to grow in size. So this is also a good age to introduce breathing exercises, such as Calming breath (see page 106) and synchronizing the breath with the yoga movements.

Enjoying the poses

It is important not to insist on children doing perfect poses or to be over-critical of their performance, as children can become easily dispirited. Try to create a joyful atmosphere in your yoga session and encourage an energetic balance between excitement and attentiveness. Assess the children's energy level. If they have loads of energy and are very restless, then get them to practice some calming exercises, such as concentration and breathing. If the children are bored or have a lack of energy, then get them doing some dynamic poses such as the Salute to the moon series (see pages 85–87) to liven them up. When yoga is practiced regularly, it can help children regulate their own energy, which can really assist them when they are going through stressful periods at school. The concentration and breathing exercises can focus their minds, and the different poses can release any pent-up tension so that they can be more relaxed when taking any tests or examinations.

Brain power

As was mentioned in the last chapter, the brain is split into two hemispheres: the left and the right. The left side is logical and rational, while the right side is intuitive and creative. The learning a child does at school mainly develops the left hemisphere: the logical, rational, and linear aspects of the mind. Creative activities, such as movement, dance, physical education, and art, are being reduced or taken out of the curriculum, so the right side of the brain is not getting the same kind of development. In yoga, both hemispheres of the brain are believed to be equally important for the complete and balanced development of a child. In a recent study, researchers looked at the effects of meditation, breathing, exercise, and biofeedback techniques on the brain. They found that when the mind was unified and relaxed, knowledge was assimilated by the brain at a deeper subconscious level and the powers of learning were accelerated. When children practice yoga, therefore, it can help them achieve their highest potential.

A holistic experience

Try to make each yoga session a holistic learning experience by involving all the senses. Let the children appreciate the touch of a soft blanket during relaxation. Burn some aromatic essential oils to stimulate their sense of smell, and bring in some visual input such as a yantra, which is a geometric diagram used in India for arresting and calming the mind (photocopy one from a book). During relaxation encourage older children to observe the sounds around them such as the birds singing or a plane flying overhead. This will help them to sharpen their hearing and awareness. Let older and more experienced children teach poses to their younger siblings, so that they improve their performance and learn tolerance and patience. Working with children in a circle or getting them to practice poses in pairs can also help to develop a positive group mentality.

Older children have a longer attention span and more stamina and endurance to attempt poses such as Candle pose (see page 75).

Getting started

This chapter covers some important points that you need to know as parents when doing yoga at home with your children. Encourage your children to stay focused as they do the poses, so that they do not become too over-excited. Calm them at the start with a simple relaxation exercise (see page 115), followed by a group exercise such as Blossoming lotus (see page 98) to get them working together. If you are a parent who is new to yoga, take a few classes yourself with a qualified yoga teacher before you start practicing with your children at home.

Before starting your yoga session, make sure there is enough space to move. Check that you have all equipment or accompaniments at hand so that your children enjoy a fun yoga session.

Where to practice

- Create a clean open space, either inside or out, for your yoga session. This space needs to be clear of any sharp objects, furniture, china, or breakables.
- Make sure it is a peaceful space, away from distractions, such as a television, telephones, or other people. Check that the temperature is warm, and pull down any blinds to avoid direct sunlight.

What to wear

- Loose, comfy, or stretchy clothing is the best to wear (see right). Avoid too-baggy outfits, or you can get caught in rolls of fabric while practicing.
- Practice in bare feet; but if any child has a wart, ask them to practice in their socks.
- Remove any watches, jewelry, or eye glasses. If a child is uncomfortable without eye glasses, then let her wear them, but remove them during upside-down poses.

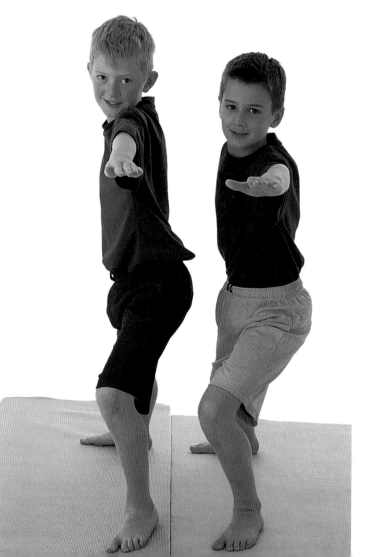

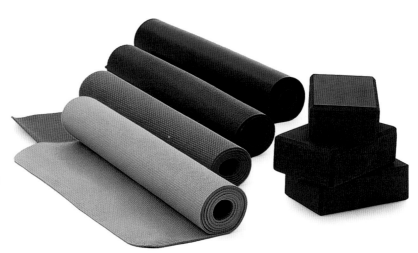

Equipment

- The best surfaces to practice yoga on are a sticky yoga mat, a rug, or a towel.
- Yoga blocks can be handy in case any poses need to be modified, or if a child requires assistance.

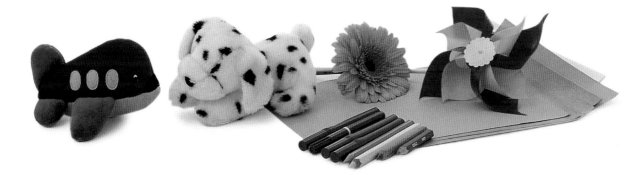

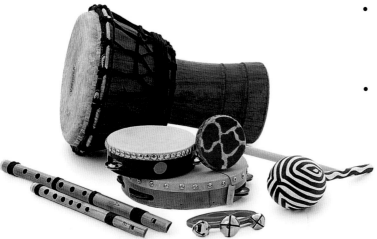

- Use additional props, such as the beanie toys in the breathing exercises (see page 105), the flower or shell for the concentration exercises (see page 112), plus paper and crayons for drawing after visualization (see page 112).
- Lively chanting and singing sessions (see page 113) will need some musical instruments, such as tambourines, rattles, and drums.

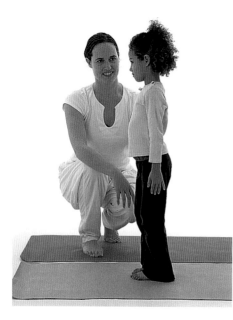

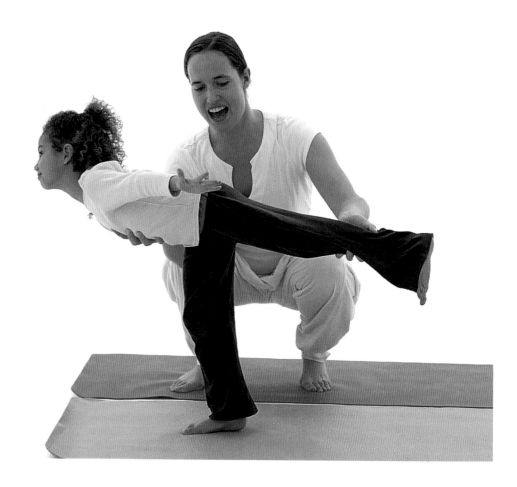

When your children are practicing the poses, always be there to help them into position. Only let them hold the pose briefly, and do not let them over-stretch at any time.

When to do yoga

- Allow at least two hours after a meal before practicing yoga. Children may want to eat during a yoga session (the poses fire up the appetite), but restrict any snacking until the end of a class, as it may cause indigestion.
- Begin with a 15-minute yoga session, building up to 20 minutes. Try to do these sessions regularly, about two to three times a week, to build up a regular routine.

How to practice yoga safely

- Always do some warm-up stretches first for about 5–10 minutes (see Chapter 2) and then work through easy poses, intermediate, and more advanced poses, but make them fun and enjoyable to do.
- You can also use the well-planned programs designed for older and younger children at the back of the book (see pages 116–127).
- Finish the session with simpler poses, breathing or concentration exercises, and a period of relaxation (see Chapter 7 and 8), so that the children leave feeling relaxed rather than over-excited.
- *Asana* means comfortable or steady seat, so it is important that a child never strains his muscles in a pose or pushes beyond his limit.
- Watch for any signs that a child is holding her breath or tensing up during a pose and tell her to keep breathing and to relax.
- Yoga breathing is always through the nose, unless the nose is blocked.
- Try and encourage children to laugh in a session, as it relieves nervous tension.
- If a child complains of a pain in any pose, make him stop performing the exercise immediately.
- Let a child rest at any point during a class in *advasana* (lying on her

tummy), Yogic sleep (lying on her back, see page 115), or Child's pose (crouched forward with arms by the side, see page 74).

- After practicing back-bending poses such as the Bow and Wheel, show the children how to do a simple forward bend such as Child's pose to release any back tension. With forward-bending poses, such as Jack knife, let them do a simple back bend such as Table pose (see page 66) to release any spinal tension.

- Candle pose and Fish pose (see pages 75 and 59) can tense the neck and shoulders, so let the children roll their heads gently from side to side to ease this.

- To avoid any injuries, encourage children to move from one pose to the next slowly and carefully.

- Children are unable to hold a pose for as long as adults, so get them to practice a pose for less time, then repeat it. This keeps them from trying to balance too long in the different positions.

- Many children have open, flexible joints or they can be double-jointed, so get them to keep their joints slightly bent so that they build up muscle, rather than over-extending a joint.

- In all the poses, show the children how to elongate their spines, rather than compress them.

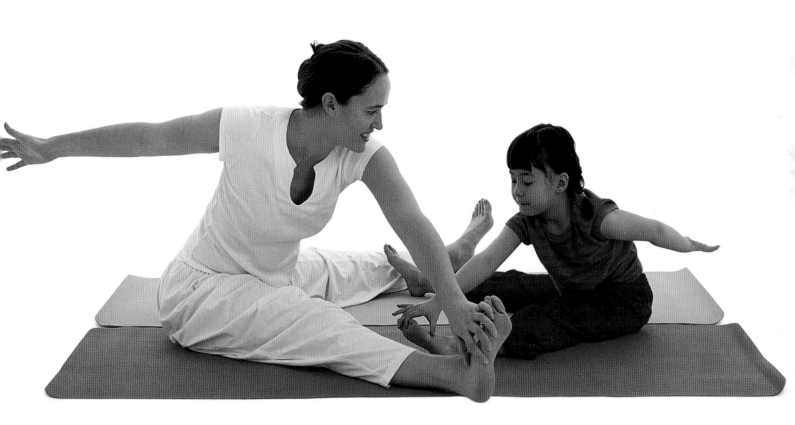

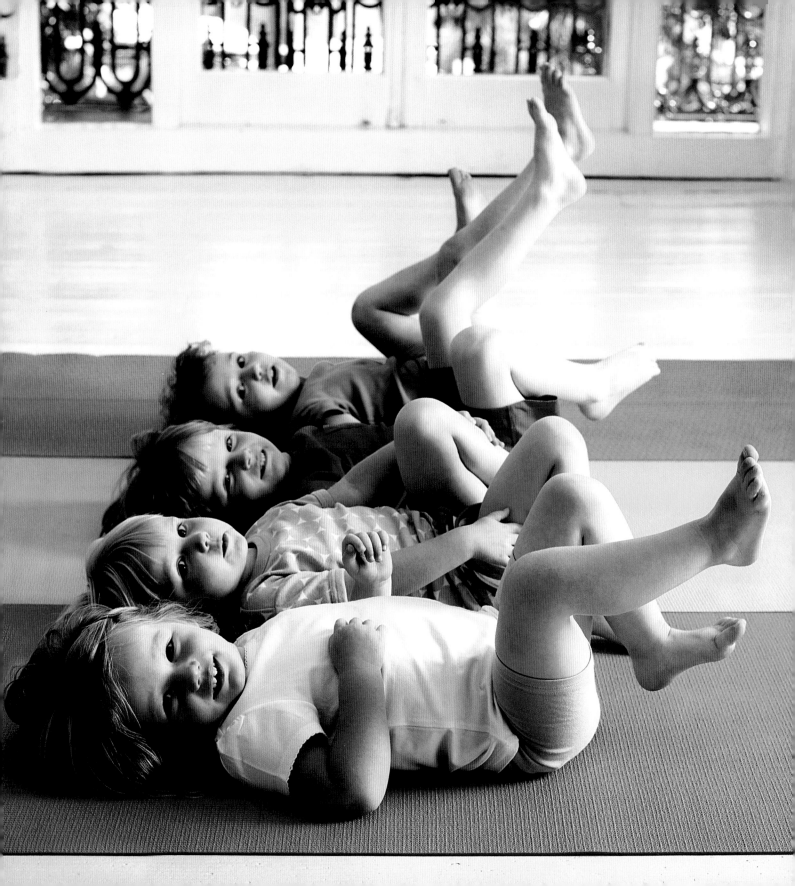

Chapter 2
Warming Up

The following exercises help to warm up the body so that children feel ready to start the yoga session. Practicing these simple movements for 5–10 minutes before they start the poses loosens the major joints of the body and warms up cold muscles, preventing injuries from occurring. Make sure they never try to force a joint in the opposite direction or to over-stretch a muscle.

Make it an enjoyable session: you can even sing the anatomy song together, "The ankle bone is connected to the knee bone, the knee bone is connected to the thigh bone," so that the children understand what they are doing.

Jiggling

To warm up the whole body and to release the joints and any pent-up nervous energy before your yoga session, do this exercise. To make it more fun, do the jiggling to music.

Stand on your mat and shake your wrists to loosen them and wave your hands around. Walk in place, lifting your knees as high as you can toward your chest. Stretch one foot out and rotate the foot, then repeat with the other foot. Keep moving until you start to feel warm.

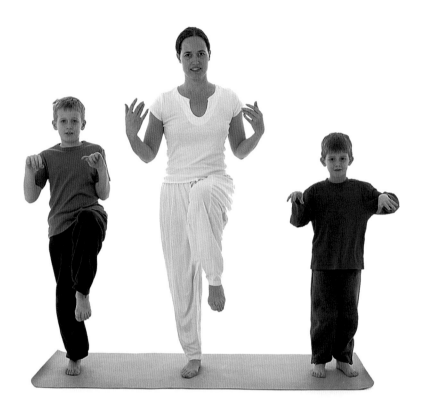

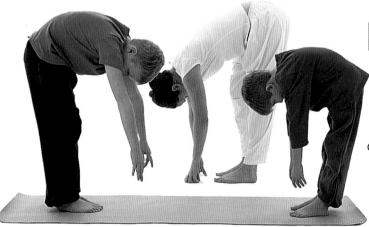

Rag doll

Yoga releases tension and promotes a feeling of relaxation during the poses. If a pose is strained, it will not have any positive effect. This warm-up helps children to relax.

Stand up straight in Mountain pose (see page 62) on your mat. Tuck your chin in toward your chest and slowly roll forward and down—try to do it one vertebra at a time. Relax your arms and neck down toward the floor, then gently shake your head up and down and from side to side. Swing gently from side to side, imagining that your upper body is like an elephant's trunk swinging in the breeze. Slowly roll up your spine, bringing your head up last. **Breath:** keep breathing evenly throughout.

Benefits
Rag doll is a relaxing forward bend that stimulates the brain, loosens the hip joints, and stretches out the spine.

Windmill circles

Warm up your upper body by imitating the action of a windmill and circling your arms backward and forward.

Stand upright on your mat in Mountain pose (see page 62) with your feet a hip-width apart.

Inhale: slowly circle your arms up and over the head, keeping your shoulders relaxed.

Exhale: continue circling all the way around, allowing your arms to move naturally out to the sides and behind you, until you are back in the start position. Repeat about twice in one direction and twice in the opposite direction. Make the circling smooth and fluid, like a working windmill. Children can have some fun trying to rotate their arms in different directions.

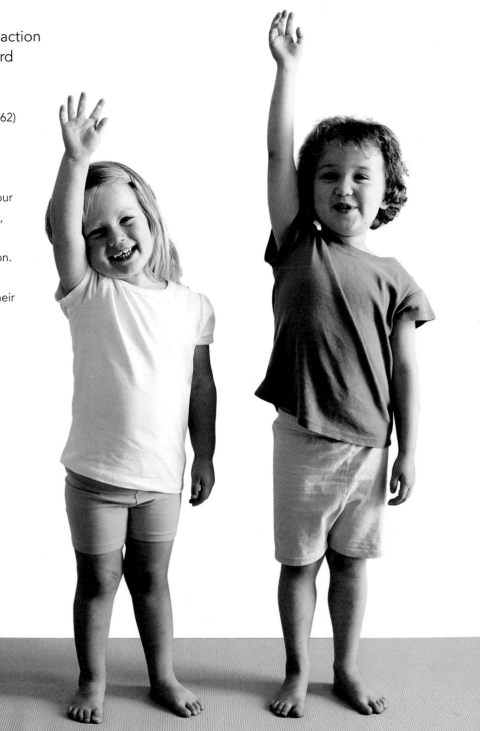

Benefits

Arm circles lubricate the shoulder joint and ease any stiffness that is felt in the upper back and neck.

Head rolls

The head is very heavy, and makes up an eighth of the entire body weight. Head rolls are a great way to loosen up tight muscles in young necks and shoulders.

1 Sit upright in a cross-legged position on your mat, with relaxed shoulders and your arms resting on your knees.

Inhale: looking ahead, tuck in your chin slightly, extend the back of the neck, and lower your right ear toward your right shoulder. Hold for a few seconds, then **exhale** and release your head back to the center.

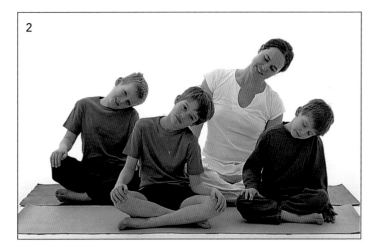

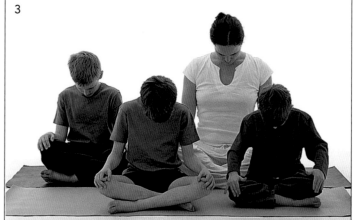

2 Inhale: roll your head, lowering your left ear toward your left shoulder. Hold for a few seconds, then **exhale** and release back to the center.

3 Inhale: tuck in your chin and roll your head forward toward your chest, keeping your back and shoulders straight. Hold for a few seconds, then **exhale** and release back to the center.

Side arm stretch

1 Sit cross-legged on your mat. Place your left palm on the floor, about 1 ft/30 cm from your hips with the fingers pointing away. **Inhale:** stretch your right arm out to the side and rotate it so that your palm is facing the ceiling. **Exhale:** stretch over to your left side with your arm close to your right ear. Bend your left elbow in as you stretch over. Hold briefly, then release back to the center.

2 Now repeat the stretch on the other side, and reach over to the right with your left arm.

Benefits

This stretch limbers up the spine and flexes the muscles of the rib cage, which helps you to breathe more easily.

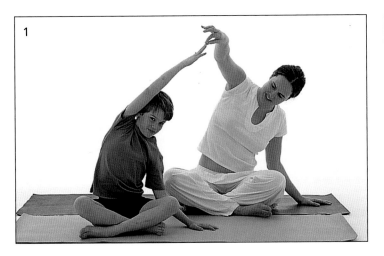

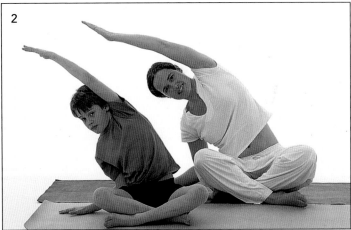

Shoulder shrugs

Shrugging the shoulders releases any tension in the upper back, neck, and shoulder muscles.

Sit cross-legged on your mat. **Inhale:** relax your arms and lift both shoulders up toward your ears.
Exhale: release them down again. Repeat several times.

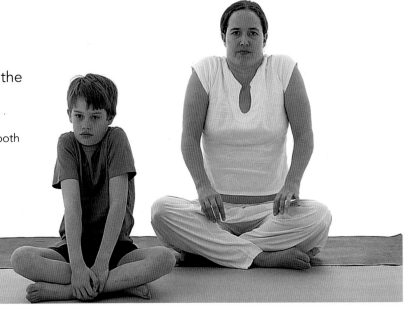

Sitting palm stretch

1 Sit cross-legged on your mat.
Inhale: interlock your fingers, turn the palms away, and stretch your arms.

2 With your arms stretched out and your elbows straight, lift up, stretching to shoulder height to loosen your upper back.

3 **Exhale:** stretch your arms over your head and open your palms toward the ceiling, keeping your neck and shoulders relaxed. Stretch both sides of your upper body evenly. Hold briefly, then release.

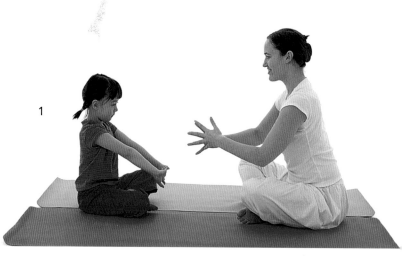

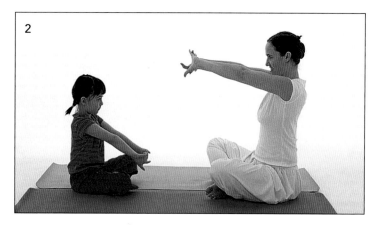

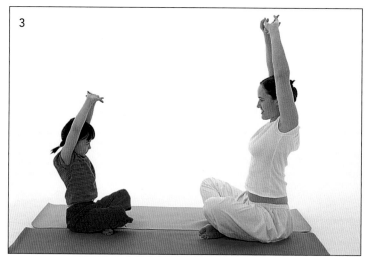

Foot rotations

This warm-up stimulates the thousands of nerve endings in your feet, benefiting your whole body. You may even feel them "buzzing" after this exercise.

Sit on your mat with your legs stretched out in front of you. Place your hands on the floor just behind your buttocks for support. Circle one foot at a time. Imagine that you are drawing circles in mid-air with your foot. Circle each foot in one direction and then the other. Repeat several times.

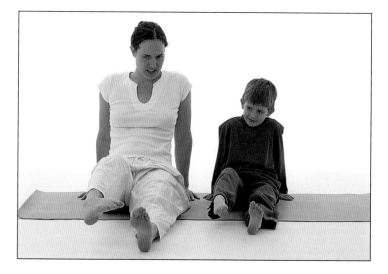

Leg stretches

Your leg muscles support the weight of your body, so doing this warm-up stretch will help keep them strong and toned. Make this stretch more enjoyable by doing it with a partner.

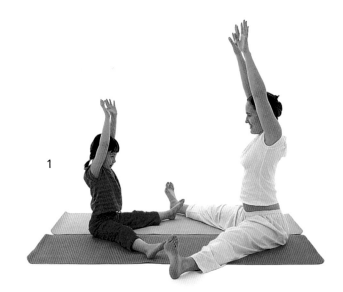

1

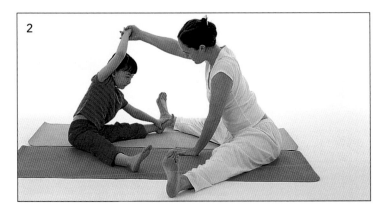

2

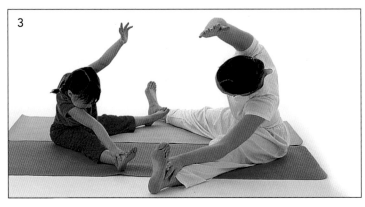

3

4

1 Sit with a straight back on your mat with your legs stretched out to each side. Point your toes upward.
Inhale: stretch your arms up over your head with your palms facing out, and reach up and stretch out your spine.

2 **Exhale:** lean sideways and hold your left foot or ankle with your hand. Stretch your right arm out and up, alongside your right ear. Stretch the right side of your torso and extend your left hand toward your left foot, keeping your torso pointing forward. Hold for a few seconds, then return to the center.

3 Repeat the movement by stretching your arm over to your right side in the same way as in Step 2.

4 **Inhale:** lean forward and place your hands on the floor in front of you. Stretch out your spine and slowly lean forward.

5 **Exhale:** bend as far forward as is comfortable and move your forehead toward the floor.

5

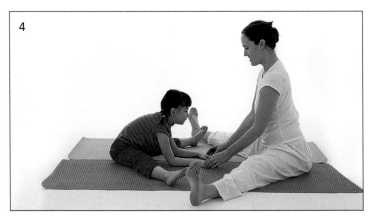

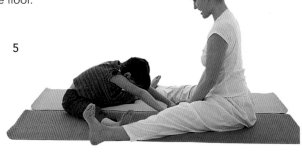

Knee to chest

This warm-up is fun to do, especially as a group, and works on the back and leg muscles while you are lying down.

1 Lie flat on your back on your mat with your feet together.

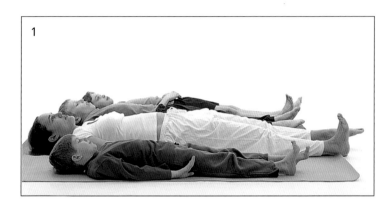

1

2 **Inhale:** raise your left leg and bend your knee. Hug your bent leg close to your chest. Keep your right leg straight by pushing into your right heel.
Exhale: try to push your lower back down toward the floor. Relax your head and neck and release any tension in your jaw. Hold briefly, then repeat with your opposite leg.

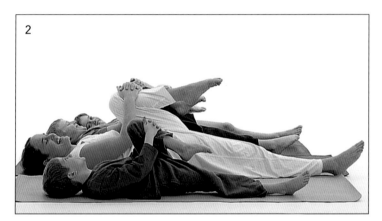

2

3 **Inhale:** raise both your legs and bend your knees toward your chest. Keep them together, hold your shins, and hug both knees tightly to your chest. Try to keep your head and lower back in contact with the floor. Hold for a few moments.
Exhale: release the hug, and hold the tops of your knees lightly with both hands. Circle your knees in one direction and then the other to gently massage the sacrum at the bottom of the back.

3

Benefits

Knee hugs lengthen the spine and increase the flexibility in your hips. Pushing your thighs against the pelvis massages your intestines and stimulates digestion.

Happy baby

This pose will make you laugh: it imitates how babies love to play with their toes and feet in their cribs.

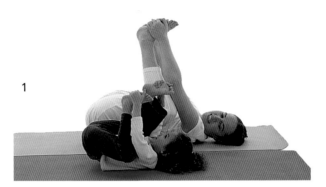

1 Lie flat on your back on a mat with your feet together.
Inhale: raise both your legs and bend your knees. Take hold of the soles of your feet with your hands.

2 Separate your knees.
Exhale: pull the soles of your feet toward you and extend your knees toward the floor beside each armpit. Gently roll from side to side.

3 Touch the soles of your feet together and pull your feet toward your head. Lift your head and gently try to touch it to your feet.

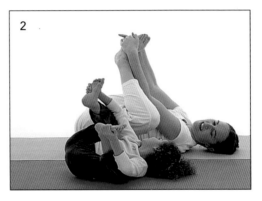

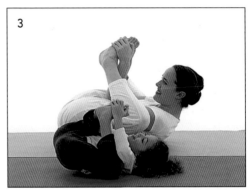

Cross-legged side twist

Sit cross-legged on your mat.
Inhale: gently turn to your right side, placing your left hand on your right knee.
Exhale: place your right hand on the floor behind you, and use your hands to twist your torso. Keep your spine straight. Hold for a few moments and then release the pose and repeat on the other side.

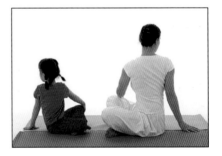

Benefits
Sitting side twist gently warms the body and makes the spine supple.

Sitting on a stool, side twist

Sitting on a stool to do this simple twist helps to keep your spine straight and elongated while you twist from side to side.

1 Sit on a small stool and place your feet and knees a hip-width apart. Rest both your hands on your knees.

2 **Inhale:** gently rotate to the right and place the back of your left hand on the outside of your right knee. Hold the back of the stool with your right hand.

Exhale: deepen the spinal twist by pressing against the outside of your right knee and pulling against the stool with your right hand. Initiate the twist from the base of your spine, turning in your hips, waist, chest, and finally your shoulders as you look over your right shoulder. Keep your neck and shoulders relaxed. Hold briefly, then come back to center.

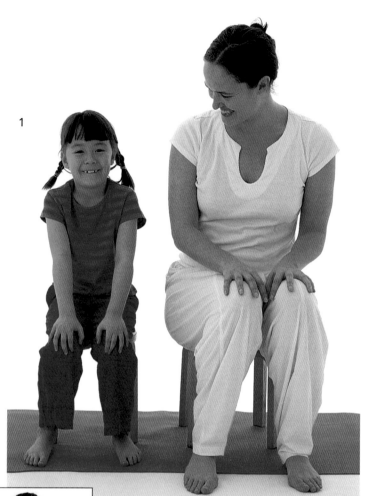

1

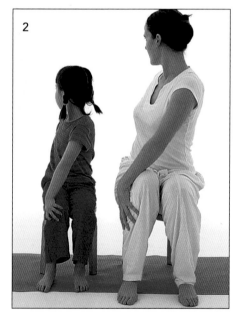

2

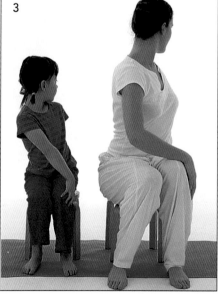

3

3 Now turn to the left and gently repeat the twist on the opposite side to balance out the body.

Lying side twist

Lying down releases any pressure on your spine, which helps you to perform this twisting movement.

1 Lie flat on your back on your mat with your arms by your sides and your knees bent.

2 **Inhale:** bend both your knees in toward your chest. Stretch your arms out to the sides with your palms facing the floor. Relax your face.

3 **Exhale:** drop your knees over to your right side, twisting from your waist. Keep your left shoulder down on the floor. Turn your head to look over to your left shoulder. Relax your neck and release your back. Hold briefly, then bring your legs back to center.

4 Now drop your knees over to your left side and repeat the twist on that side.

Benefits

This warm-up is very good if your back feels a bit sore or painful.

1

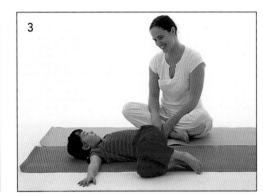

2

3

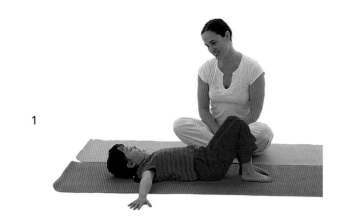

4

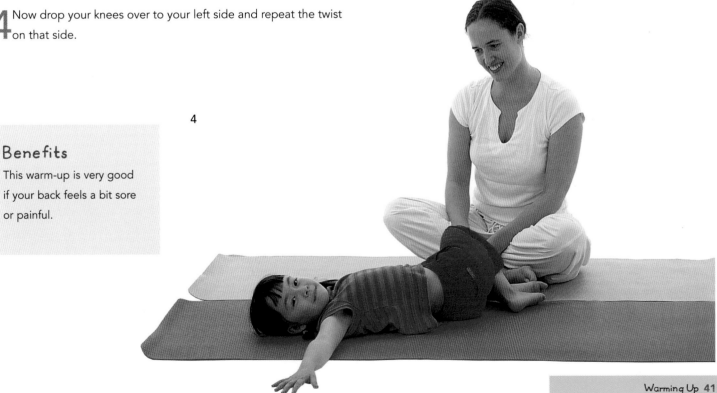

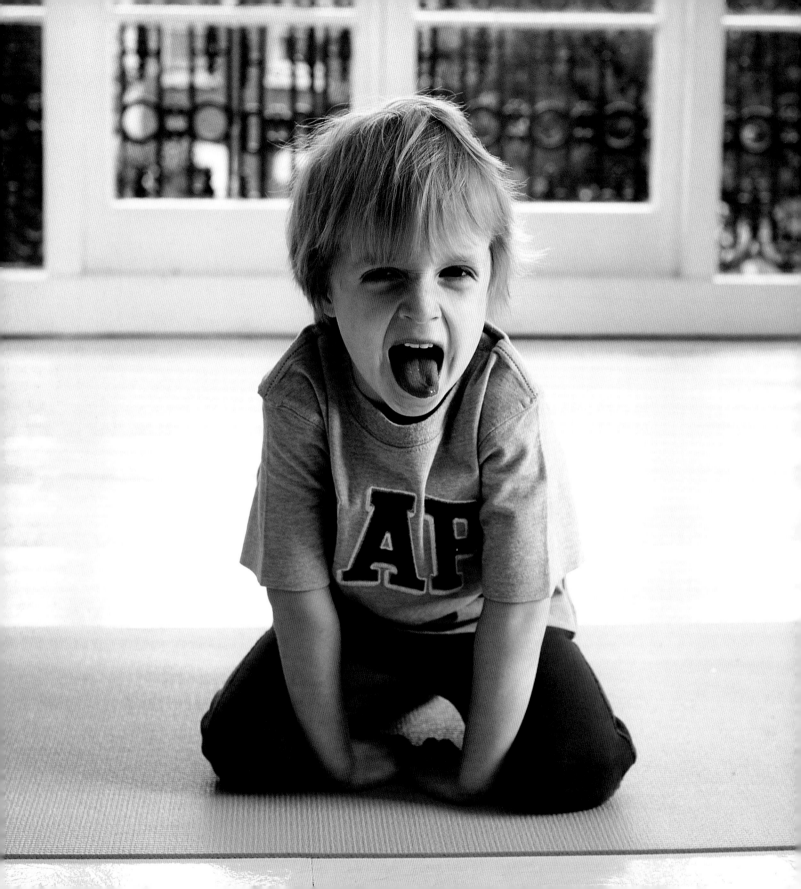

Chapter 3
Animal Poses

Children love animals. They enjoy going to the zoo and to the farm to see and pet all the different creatures. What better way to increase a child's knowledge of the animal kingdom than for them to get down on all fours and imitate a cat, for example? Let your children watch a family pet, and see how it eats, moves, stretches, and rests. Let them listen to the sounds it makes and then see if they can imitate it.

Use these poses creatively in an enjoyable yoga session that young children, particularly, will love. Make up animal stories that can imitate or describe an imaginary trip to the zoo or farm.

Downward dog pose

Dogs are one of our oldest companions. They are loyal, playful, and very loving pets. There is a lot we can learn from a dog. Have you ever watched a dog stretch itself after a nap? Here is what it feels like.

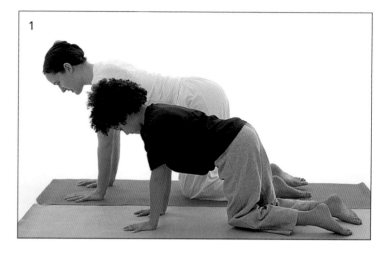

1 Kneel on all fours on your mat and place your hands underneath your shoulders, with your knees underneath your hips.

2 **Inhale:** tuck your toes under, push into the palms of your hands, raise your hips up and back, lengthening your spine.
Exhale: straighten your arms, and the backs of your knees, and stretch your heels toward the floor. Look back between your feet.
Breath: keep breathing evenly. Take a long, deep stretch and then rest back on all fours.

CHILD'S TIP
Feel free to make any doggy noises such as barking or whimpering when you are in Dog pose.

Benefits
Dog pose strengthens the arms and legs, and sends a fresh supply of blood to the head. It can help to correct curvature of the spine.

2

Cat pose

Cats are agile, flexible, and graceful. Learn the secret of how you can stay supple from the cat. Cats know how to get plenty of rest and stay warm and cozy, so their muscles do not get stiff.

1 Start on all fours like a cat on your mat. Place your hands directly below your shoulders and spread out your fingers. Keep your knees in line with your hips and your toes pointing backward.

2 **Inhale:** lift your tailbone up toward the ceiling so that your lower back becomes concave in shape. As you do this movement, your head will lift up naturally toward the ceiling.

3 **Exhale:** arch your back and roll your head down toward your chest. Stretch your spine as high as you can and tuck your tailbone under. Tuck your head in, pointing your chin toward your chest. Repeat Steps 2 and 3 several times or until you get tired. Make the movements as fluid as possible.

When you are in Step 3, see how high you can lift your spine, feeling the pull on your tummy muscles. With practice, and as you become more supple, this will get much easier to perform.

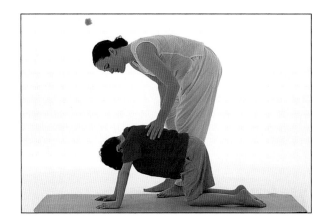

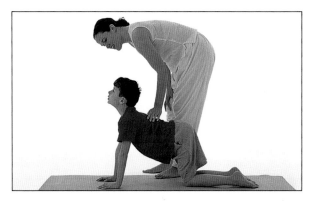

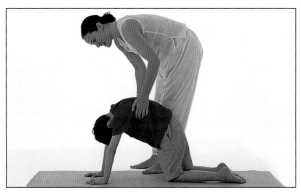

PARENT'S TIP
If a child becomes tired doing this pose, let him relax into Child's pose (see page 74) and rest for a few moments before repeating the exercise.

Tiger pose

Tigers are like bigger, stronger cats, but are much fiercer hunters.

1 Start on all fours like a tiger on your mat. Place your hands underneath your shoulders and your knees so that they are underneath your hips.

2 **Inhale:** arch your back and roll your head down toward your chest. Stretch your spine high and bend your right knee toward your chest. See if you can touch your head with your knee.

3 **Exhale:** drop your tummy toward the floor. Press your hands into the floor and lift up your chest and head. Simultaneously, kick your right leg up and back. Keep your knee bent and point your toes toward your head. Repeat Steps 2 and 3 with your left leg. Make all the movements as fluid as possible. Rest forward in Child's pose (see page 74).

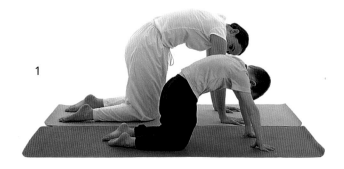

Benefits

Tiger pose tones the spine and increases flexibility in the hips. It also strengthens the thigh and buttock muscles.

Lion pose

Lions are another member of the feline family, along with cats and tigers. A lion's roar can be heard up to 5 miles/8 km away. Let us learn to roar like a lion.

Sit on your heels on your mat with your knees apart. Place your hands on the floor with your fingertips facing toward your body. Lean forward, resting your body on your arms.
Inhale: tilt your head back.
Exhale: stick out your tongue and roar loudly like a lion. Repeat 2–6 times.

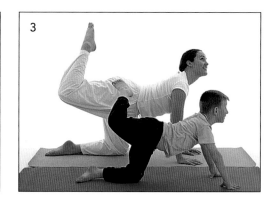

Cow face pose

Cows in India are sacred, and they are revered for their patience and tolerance. They also nourish us with their milk. This pose is called Cow face because the shape of the knees makes a cow face, with the feet as the horns.

1 Sit on your mat with your legs straight out. Bend your knees and place the soles of your feet on the floor.

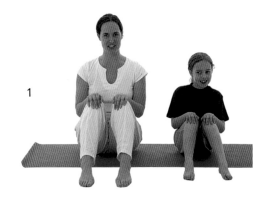

2 **Inhale:** bend your left leg and pass it under your right leg so that your knee is in line with the center of your body. Place your heel on the floor next to your right hip.

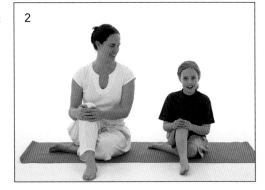

3 **Exhale:** bend your right leg over your left so that the heel is in line with your left hip. The knees should be stacked on top of each other.

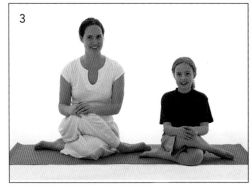

4 **Inhale:** raise your right arm in the air and stretch up as tall as you can.

5 **Exhale:** bend your right elbow and reach your right hand behind the back of your neck. Bend your left arm behind your back at waist level. Join the fingers of each hand behind your back, if you can. Keep your head and neck straight.

Breath: keep breathing evenly and hold the pose for as long as is comfortable. Repeat the steps with the opposite arm and leg.

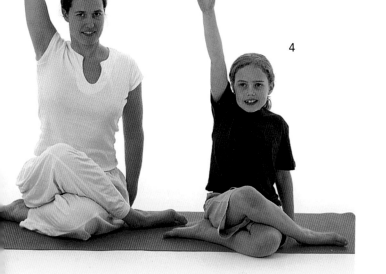

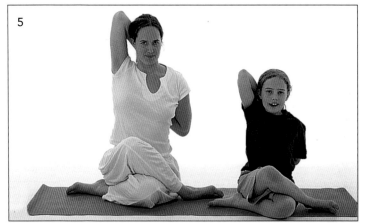

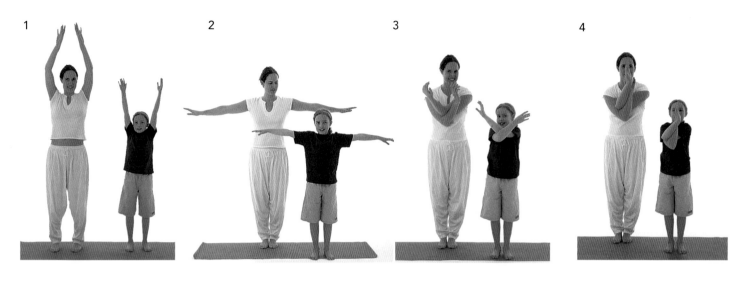

Eagle pose

Eagles can spy their prey from miles away with their powers of concentration. So practice Eagle pose to gain focus and balance. It can be difficult to master, but it is well worth it.

1 Stand up straight in Mountain pose (see page 62).
Inhale: focus your gaze on a spot in front of you to help you balance, then raise your arms above your head.

2 Release your arms in a circular motion out to the sides and start to wrap your right arm underneath your left.

3 **Exhale:** twist your arms around each other and get them into position to touch your palms.

4 Bend your elbows so that your palms are together in front of your nose.

5 **Inhale:** bend your knees slightly and lift your left thigh over your right thigh.

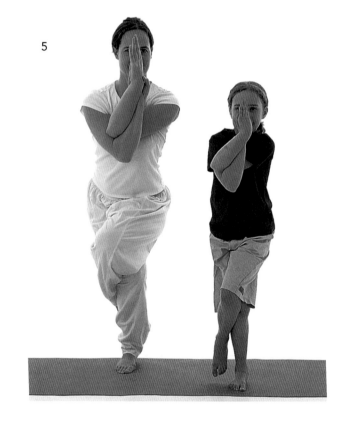

Exhale: wrap your left foot around your right calf. Try to keep your knees and elbows in one line in the center of the body. Hold briefly, then release and repeat on the other side.

Pigeon pose

Pigeons have a very intelligent homing instinct and are used to carry messages over long distances. The proud, puffed-up chest of the pigeon forms the main part of performing this pose.

Benefits

Pigeon pose tones the neck and shoulders and increases blood flow to the lower spine. It stimulates the functioning of the thyroid, parathyroid, adrenals, and reproductive glands.

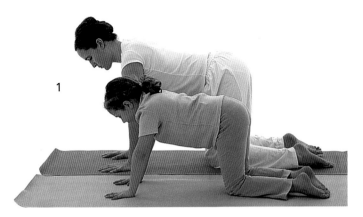

1 Start on all fours on your mat. Place your hands underneath your shoulders and your knees underneath your hips.

2 **Inhale:** slide your right knee forward between your hands. Slide your left leg straight back, until your left hip and right heel are in line.

Exhale: press into your hands and lift and puff up your chest. Look up, rolling your shoulders down and arching your back. Keep stretching the left leg back. Hold briefly, then release and repeat on the opposite side.

3 Release the pose and rest forward in Child's pose to relax any tension in your lower back.

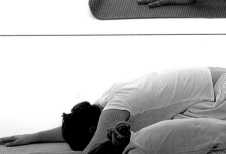

Monkey

This pose is more commonly known as a split. The pose imitates the monkey's ability to reach from one tree to the next and to swing long distances with its arms.

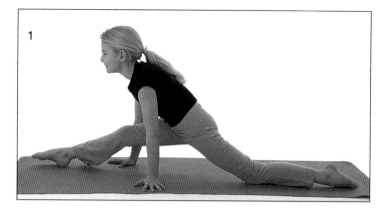

1 Start from a kneeling position on your mat.
Inhale: extend your right leg forward with your heel touching the floor. Lean forward slightly and place the palms of your hands on the floor on either side of your outstretched leg.

2 **Exhale:** slowly slide your right leg forward and your left leg straight back until you reach a full split. Alternatively, go as far as is possible. If you are comfortable, lift both your arms over your head and reach up. Stay in this position briefly, then release and repeat with your other leg.

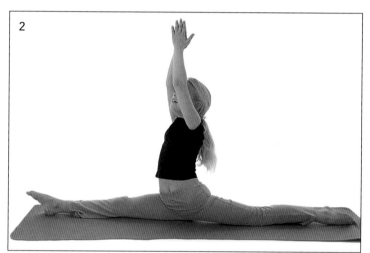

Camel pose

Camels are known as the "ships of the desert," as they store water in their humps, letting them go for days without drinking. This enables them to carry people and supplies for miles across the desert. Experience how it feels to be a camel.

Start from a kneeling position on your mat.
Inhale: lift your body up off your heels so that you are balancing on your knees. Place your knees a hip-width apart and point your toes.
Exhale: lift up your chest into the shape of a camel's hump and look back. Reach right back and take hold of each ankle with your hands. Keep arching your back, lifting your chest, and gently pushing your hips forward. Hold the stretch for a few seconds, then support your lower back with your hands and slowly come back into an upright position.

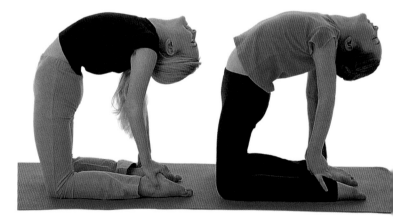

Frog pose

Frogs are amphibians, living both in water and on land. They have big strong back legs so they can leap from one lily pad to the next. See how high you can jump.

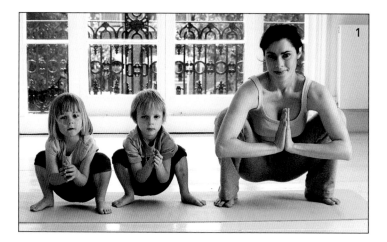

1 Stand with your feet a hip-width apart on your mat.
Inhale: balancing on your feet, squat down and reach toward the ground. Bring your hands into prayer position—*namaste*—in front of your chest. You can press your knees out to the sides with your elbows to increase the stretch in your hips.
Hold briefly.

2 **Exhale:** leap as high in the air as you can, like a frog.
Repeat the pose several times, seeing how high you can jump.

Benefits

Frog pose tones the abdominal organs and relieves any aches or pains in the back.

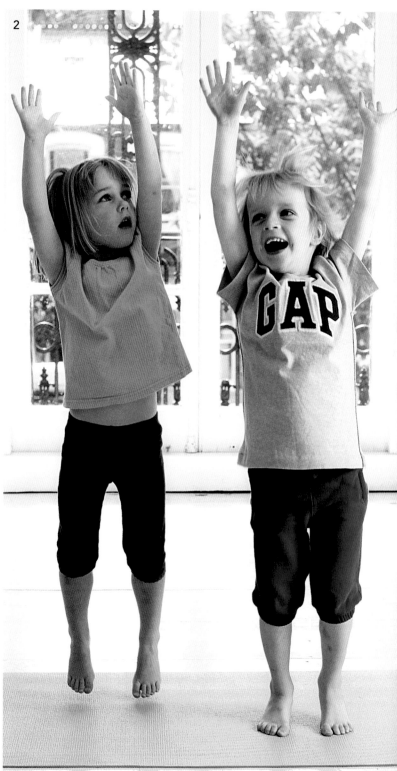

Crow pose

Crows are intelligent. Their black color means that they can easily recognize each other, and it protects them from predators at night. Turn your arms into two crow's legs to perform the pose. Learn this pose in a yoga class before practicing at home.

1

PARENT'S TIP
Place a pillow on the floor in front of your child's head in case she loses her balance and starts to roll forward.

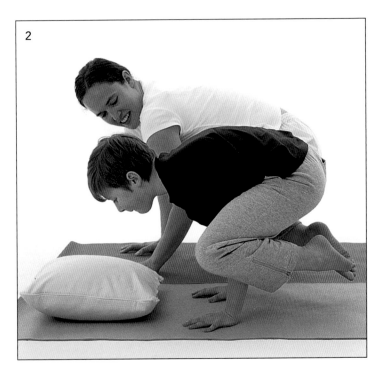

2

1 Squat down on your mat and place your hands on the floor in front of you, a shoulder-width apart. Spread your fingers wide to make two crow's feet.
Inhale: bend your elbows back and rest your shins on your upper arms, with your knees close to your armpits.

2 **Exhale:** shift your body weight forward and lift your feet off the floor. Keep your head up, and look forward, or you may roll right over. Hold briefly, then release.

Benefits
Crow pose strengthens your arms and wrists, and improves your concentration.

Cobra pose

Cobras are venomous snakes that use their super-strong spines to slither across the ground and even climb trees. When a cobra is threatened or about to attack it will hiss, rear up, and flatten its neck ribs into a hood. You can practice this position in Cobra pose.

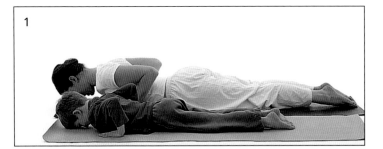

1 Lie on your tummy on your mat.
Inhale: place your hands underneath your shoulders, with your fingers pointing forward, keeping your elbows tucked in close to your chest. Extend your chin forward onto the floor. Bring your legs together to form one long cobra tail.

2 **Exhale:** slowly lift your head and chest and arch your back. Try not to place too much weight on your hands, but use your strong back muscles to lift your chest as high as possible.

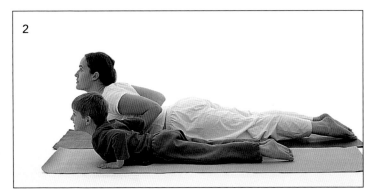

3 If Step 2 feels comfortable, then **inhale** and as you **exhale** push into your palms and lift your chest, arching your back. Look up to the ceiling. Hold briefly and hiss like a snake, then slowly come down.

3

4

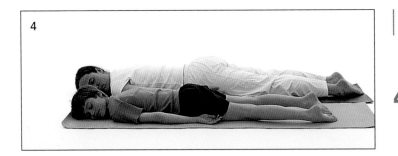

CHILD'S TIP
Hiss as loud as you like in Step 3.

4 Rest for a few moments on your tummy on your mat with your head turned to one side.

Twisting cobra pose

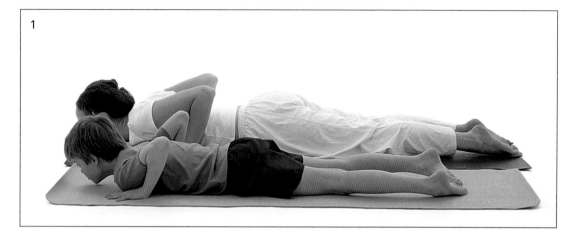

1 Lie on your tummy on your mat.

Inhale: place your hands underneath your shoulders, with your fingers pointing forward, and keep your elbows tucked in close to your chest. Extend your chin forward onto the floor. Bring your legs together to form one long cobra tail.

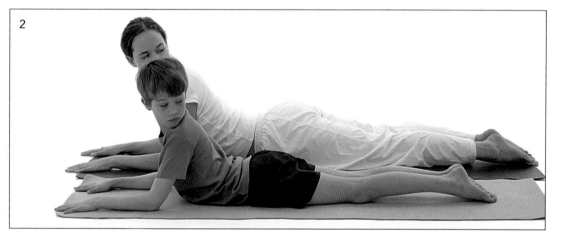

2 **Exhale:** come into Cobra pose (see page 53). Slide your hands forward until your elbows are under your shoulders. Keep your chest lifted and shoulders arching back. Turn your head to look over your left shoulder and hiss. Hold for a few moments, then release.

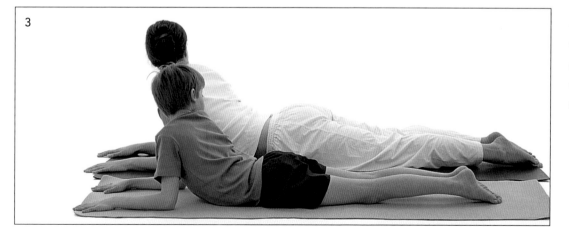

3 Repeat the movement on the opposite side, hissing over your right shoulder. Slowly come down and then release the position.

King cobra pose

The king cobra is the largest venomous snake. It can grow up to 18 ft/5.5 m long. The king cobra can smell using its forked tongue. It does not have ears, but can feel vibrations from the ground—see if you can, too.

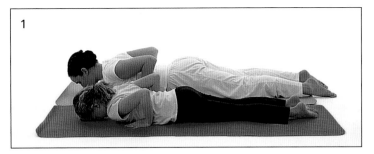

1 Lie on your tummy on your mat.
Inhale: place your hands underneath your shoulders, with your fingers pointing forward and your elbows tucked in close to your chest. Extend your chin forward onto the floor. Bring your legs together to form one long cobra tail.

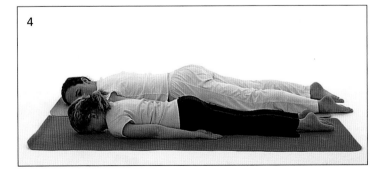

2 **Exhale:** come into Cobra pose. Separate your legs so that they are a hip-width apart. Push into your palms and stretch up, arching your back as high as you can, while looking up toward the ceiling.

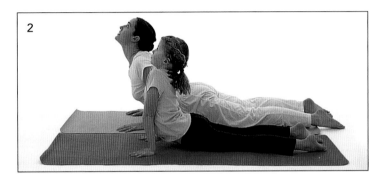

Benefits

This pose strengthens the spine and keeps it supple. The movements massage the tummy's organs and help to improve the digestion.

3 **Inhale**, then **exhale**: bend your knees and see if you can touch the crown of your head to the soles of your feet. Hold briefly, then release the pose.

4 Rest for a few moments on your tummy with your head turned to one side.

Locust pose

Locusts are similar insects to grasshoppers, and have big hind legs for jumping. Practicing Locust pose helps you to develop strong leg and lower back muscles, so that you can jump much higher.

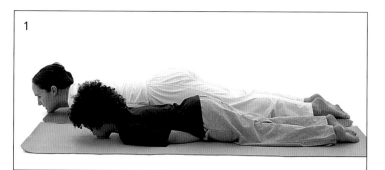

1 Lie on your tummy on your mat.
Inhale: tuck your arms underneath your body, with palms facing either up or down. Extend your chin on the floor. Bring your legs together.

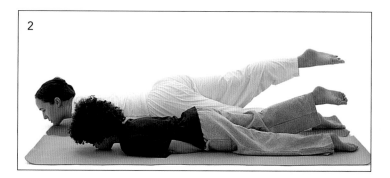

2 **Exhale:** extend your right leg and lift it up as high as you can without lifting your hip off your forearm. Hold for 10 seconds, then slowly release your leg. Repeat the movement with your left leg.

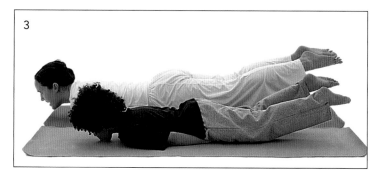

3 For a more advanced movement, try the full pose. Lie on your stomach as in Step 1.
Exhale: shift your body weight slightly forward toward your shoulders and chest. Lift up both legs simultaneously. Hold for a few seconds, then slowly release the pose.

RELEASING TENSION

After practicing a series of back bends, it is advisable to stretch the back in the opposite direction. An excellent way to release tension in the spine after back-bending is to relax in Child's pose. If you are going to practice more back-bending exercises, then simply lie on the floor either on your back or your tummy with your head turned to one side, between poses, to relax your spine.

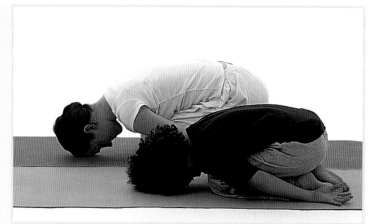

Butterfly pose

Butterflies are beautiful and delicate creatures. They bring a splash of color to the garden in the summer as they flit from flower to flower, gathering sweet nectar. See how well you can imitate them.

Sit with your legs outstretched on your mat.

Inhale: bend both knees and bring your feet in toward you as close as possible. Put the soles of your feet together.

Exhale: drop your knees out to the side. These are your butterfly wings. Hold your feet and gently flap your wings from side to side for several seconds. Keep your spine straight and lifted.

CHILD'S TIP
As you flap your butterfly wings, imagine you are in your garden at home collecting nectar from all the flowers there.

Benefits

Practicing the Butterfly pose helps to increase the mobility in your hip joints.

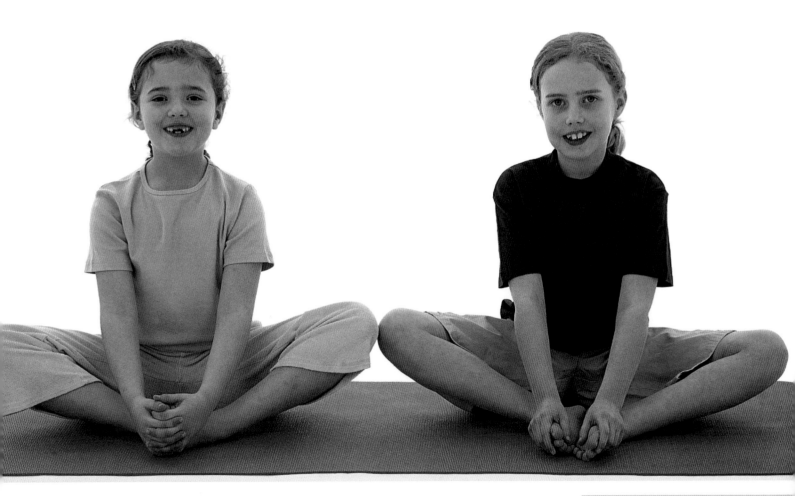

Tortoise pose

Tortoises carry their homes—their hard, bony shells—on their backs. When they get scared they hide in their shells. Learn to be like the tortoise, hiding in its home.

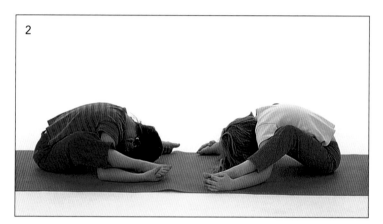

1 Sit with your legs outstretched on your mat.
Inhale: bend your knees, separate your legs, and place your feet flat on the mat, about 2 ft/60 cm away from your buttocks.

2 **Exhale:** bend forward and slide your arms underneath your knees and toward the outsides of your feet. Straighten your legs as much as possible and lean forward and touch your forehead to the floor.

3 Pretend to be a tortoise and keep peeking your head out from under your shell to say "hello" to your partner. Hold for a few moments, then release.

PARENT'S TIP
This is a great pose for children to practice in pairs.

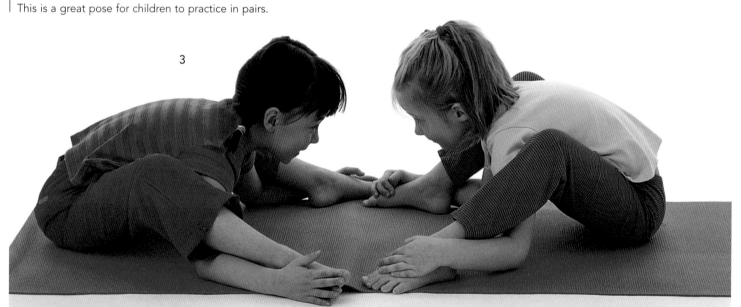

Fish pose

Fish live underwater, either in rivers and lakes or in the sea. They do not breathe oxygen through their mouths, but filter air from the water through their gills at the sides of their body. Feel how it is to be a fish in these movements.

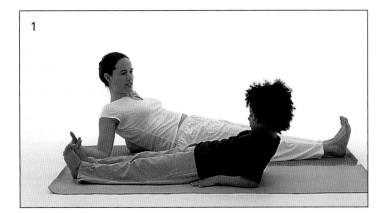

1 Lie on your back on your mat with your arms and legs together. **Inhale:** press into your elbows and lift your head and torso so that you look down at your feet.

2 **Exhale:** lift up your chest, arch your back, and place the crown of your head on the floor. Balance your body weight between your elbows and the crown of your head. Hold for a few seconds. To come out of the posture, lift up your head and slowly roll down.

2

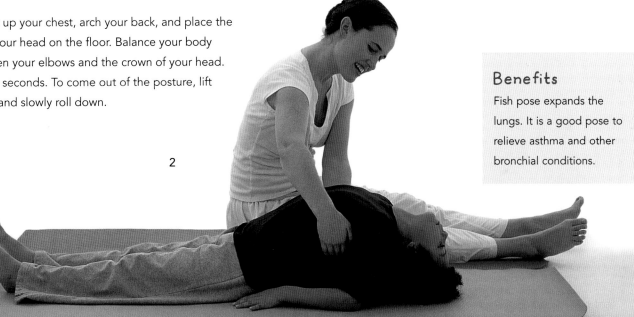

Benefits

Fish pose expands the lungs. It is a good pose to relieve asthma and other bronchial conditions.

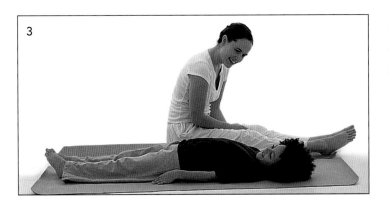

3 After an exercise that stretches your neck such as Candle pose (see page 75) and this pose, lie flat on the mat and roll your head from side to side to release any neck tension.

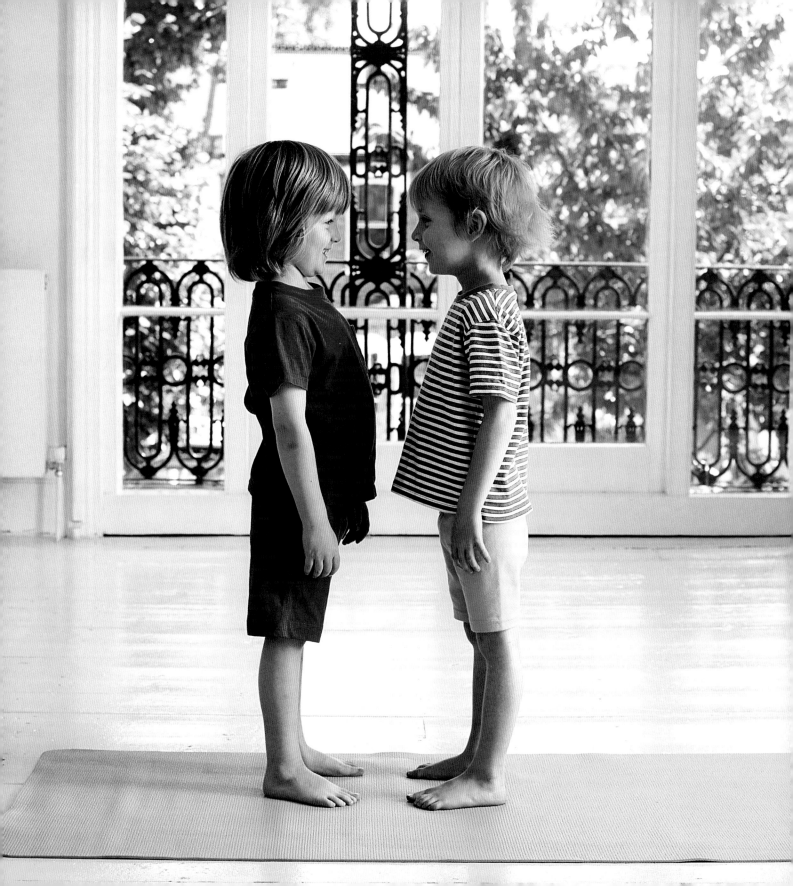

Chapter 4

Object Poses

The majority of the yoga postures in this chapter are static poses that are held without moving the body for a few seconds or more. These poses gently massage a child's internal organs, muscles, and glands. They relax the nervous system and calm the mind, so they are particularly good for very active children.

Many of these yoga poses are named after everyday objects, such as a table, boat, or teapot. Try and invent some stimulating stories that mix these poses with the animal poses in the last chapter so that the children can really get involved and have a fun yoga experience.

Mountain pose

Mountains are big, strong, steady, and still. This pose is the basic standing posture that teaches us how to stand firmly on our own two feet.

Stand upright on your mat with your feet together. Tense your thigh muscles so that your legs are solid as rock. Tuck your tailbone under, lift your chest, and stand tall. Relax your shoulders and put your arms down by your sides. Your body should be in a straight line from your ankles to the crown of your head. Stand still and steady like a mountain so that not even the strongest wind can move you.

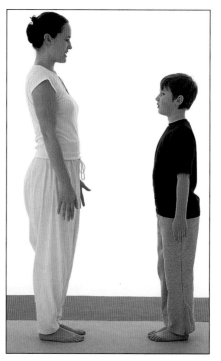

Benefits
Mountain pose gives you a good posture and focuses the mind.

Tree pose

Trees are like the lungs of the world—they clean the air and provide us with oxygen-rich air to breathe. Without trees, the earth would turn to a desert.

CHILD'S TIP
Do not worry if you wobble a bit doing this pose: trees always sway and move in the breeze.

Stand upright on your mat in Mountain pose (see above). Focus on a point on the wall in front of you to help you keep your balance. **Inhale:** take your weight into your left leg, then bend your right leg and place your right foot on the inside of your left leg anywhere between your ankle and thigh. Eventually, you want to place your foot on the top of your inner thigh.

When you are balanced on one leg and feel steady, **exhale** and raise your arms in prayer position over your head. Hold for as long as it is comfortable, then release and repeat with your other leg.

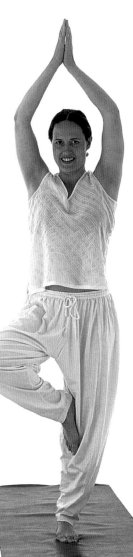

Palm tree pose

Palm trees are found in hot countries. They have long, thin ribbed trunks and big long leaves that sprout from the top of the truck. See how well you can imitate one.

Stand upright on your mat in Mountain pose (see opposite), then step your feet a hip-width apart.
Inhale: interlock your fingers and press your palms away from you.
Exhale: raise your arms above your head. Reach right up onto your "tippy" toes and stretch up as tall as you can. Hold briefly, and then release.

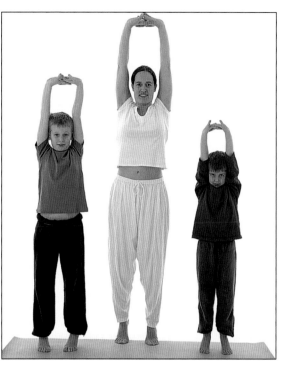

Swaying palm tree pose

Palm trees are strong and flexible and can withstand mighty winds, even hurricanes.

1 Stand upright on your mat in Mountain pose (see opposite).
Inhale: interlock your fingers and press your palms away from you.
Exhale: raise your arms above your head. Stretch up tall and lean as far as you can to the right. Hold briefly, then return to the center.

2 Stretch up tall again and then lean over to the left to stretch out the other side. Hold briefly, then return to the center. Repeat the pose a few times on both sides.

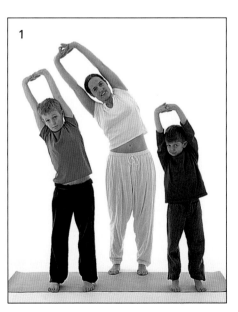

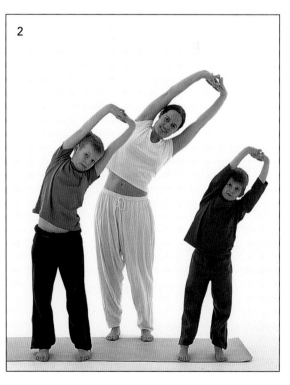

Teapot pose

This pose is a fun way to introduce preschool children to more difficult standing poses such as Triangle.

1 Stand upright on your mat in Mountain pose (see page 62). **Inhale:** step your feet about 2 ft/60 cm apart. Place your left hand on your waist to form the teapot handle. Extend your right arm to the side, with the right elbow and wrist slightly bent and the fingers pointing away from your body at shoulder height. **Exhale:** Turn your right foot out and your left foot in slightly. Keeping your arms in place, tilt your torso to the right to pour yourself a fresh cup of tea.

2 Repeat on the other side, pouring a cup on tea with your left arm.

Benefits
This pose strengthens your legs, and helps you concentrate better.

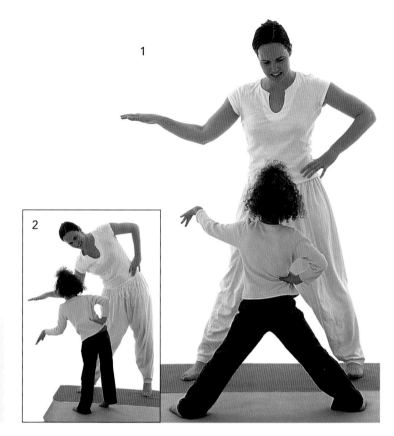

Triangle pose

Learn some geometry with yoga. Did you know that three angles form a triangle? A three-dimensional triangle is called a pyramid.

1 Stand upright on your mat in Mountain pose (see page 62), then step your feet 3 ft/1 m apart. **Inhale:** turn your left foot out and your right foot in slightly.

2 **Exhale:** bend over to the left, keeping your arms in a straight line, and place your left hand on your left leg between your ankle and thigh. Look up toward your right hand. Hold briefly, then come back to the center, and repeat on the other side.

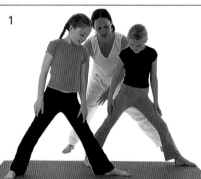

Benefits
This pose is a great stretch that tones your waist and intercostal muscles. It also stimulates the nervous system.

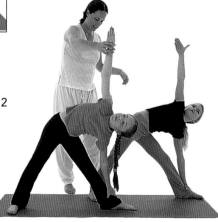

Balancing stick pose

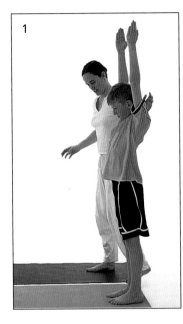

CHILD'S TIP
Be like Superman in this pose, and feel how you fly through the air.

This pose teaches coordination and balance, and increases your muscle strength.

1 Stand upright on your mat in Mountain pose (see page 62). **Inhale:** raise your arms up over your head with your palms facing and the fingers extended. Stretch up and lean slightly back.

2 **Exhale:** step your left foot forward, bend and propel your body weight forward while simultaneously lifting your back right leg off the floor. Straighten your left leg so that your body, arms, and right leg are parallel to the floor and look forward. Hold a few seconds, then come back to center and repeat on the opposite side.

Canoe pose

Canoes are small boats that were originally carved out of tree trunks. Native Americans used canoes for crossing rivers and hunting. See what it feels like to be a canoe.

1 Sit upright on your mat with your back straight and your legs stretched out in front.
Inhale: extend your arms at shoulder height with your fingers outstretched.

2 **Exhale:** slowly lower your torso backward toward the floor until it is about 6 in/15 cm away. Lift your feet until you are balancing on your buttocks. Hold briefly, then return to sitting.

Benefits
This pose strengthens your tummy muscles, and is excellent for relieving nervous tension.

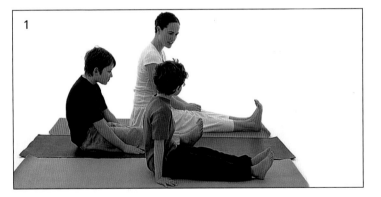

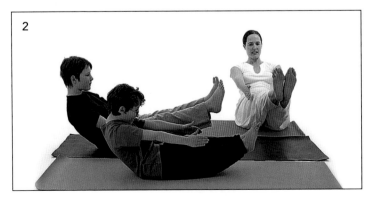

1

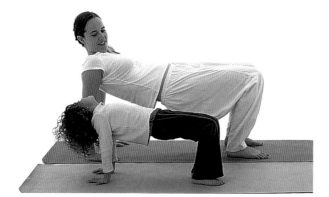

2

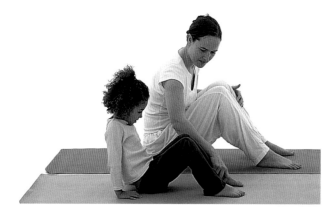

3

Table pose

To eat a meal you need both a table and a chair. In this pose you are going to be the table. Half the children can be tables, while the other half can be chairs (opposite).

1 Sit on the floor on your mat with your legs straight in front of you.
Inhale: place the palms of your hands just behind your hips. Then bend your knees, placing the soles of your feet on the floor a hip-width apart.

2 **Exhale:** press into your palms and the soles of your feet and lift your hips until your torso and thighs make a straight line. Hold briefly, and then release the pose back down.

3 For a more advanced pose after Step 1, as you **exhale**, keep your legs straight and place the palms of your hands just behind your hips. Lift your chest and hips and stretch the soles of your feet toward the floor.

Chair pose

Chairs come in many shapes and sizes. Some have high backs with hard seats, some are cushioned and cozy, others fold up. What kind of chair are you going to be?

1 Stand upright on your mat in Mountain pose (see page 62). **Inhale:** step your feet a hip-width apart. Stretch your arms out in front of you at shoulder height, keeping your fingers together.

2 **Exhale:** bend your knees and sit back and down, as if you were about to sit in a chair. Keep lifting your chest and feel the weight back on your heels. Hold briefly, then come back to center.

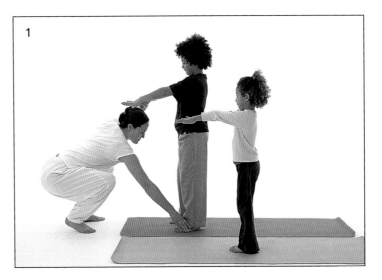

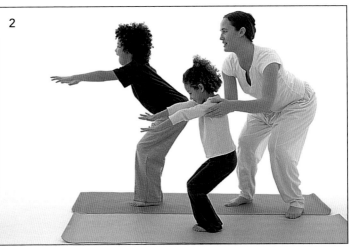

Benefits

Chair pose makes the joints more flexible, and keeps your knees and ankles healthy.

Boat pose

This pose is an upright version of Canoe (see page 65), and needs good concentration and tummy strength to perform it correctly.

1 Sit on your mat with your legs stretched out in front.
Inhale: bend your knees and place the soles of your feet on the floor about 1 ft/30 cm from your buttocks. Place your hands underneath your knees.

2 **Exhale:** slowly lean back until your feet lift right off the mat and you are balancing on your buttocks.

3 Once you are balanced, slowly straighten your knees and extend your legs. Release your hands but keep your arms lifted and stretching forward, palms facing each other. Keep your chest lifted.
Breath: keep breathing evenly. Hold for a few moments, then release the pose.

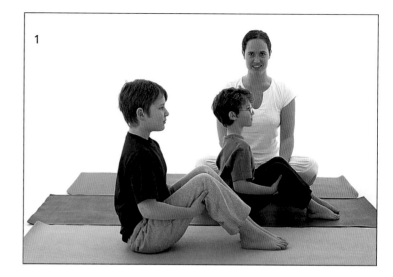

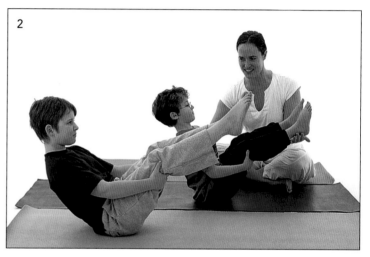

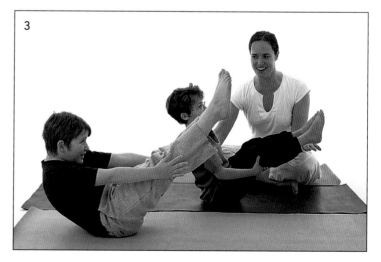

Threading the needle pose

Needlework is an essential craft that is practiced worldwide to make clothes and soft furnishings such as quilts and tapestries. See how expert you can become at "threading the needle."

1 Start on all fours on your mat, placing your hands underneath your shoulders and your knees beneath your hips.

2 **Inhale:** lift your right arm and thread it underneath your left, until your right shoulder and the right side of your face rest on the floor.

3 When your face touches the floor, **exhale**, and lift your left arm upward. Hold briefly, release back to the start position, then repeat on the other side.

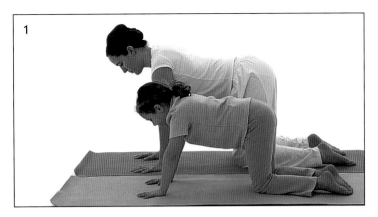

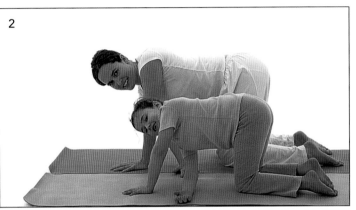

Benefits
Threading the needle pose is a gentle twist that tones and massages the spine.

3

Thunderbolt pose

Thunderbolts or lightning are bright streaks of electrical current that you can see in the sky during a storm. In yoga, thunderbolts represent flashes of inspiration or understanding. So get inspired by doing this pose.

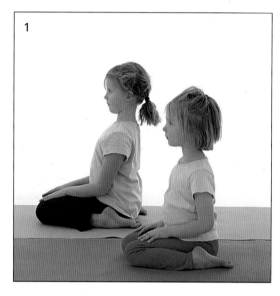

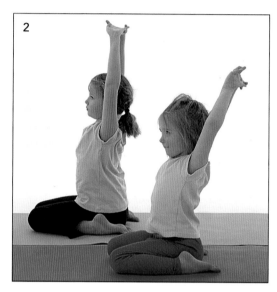

1 Kneel on your mat. Keep your knees together and spread your feet a little wider than a hip-width apart. Sit between your heels and keep your toes pointing straight back. Sit for as long as it is comfortable.

2 **Inhale:** stretch your arms up over your head and stretch out your spine. If this feels comfortable, continue to Step 3.

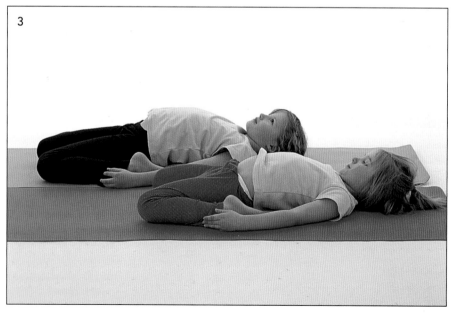

3 **Exhale:** lean back onto your elbows and slowly lower yourself to the floor. Once your shoulders and back of the head touch the floor, either keep your arms by your side or stretch them over your head.

Bridge pose

Bridges are essential constructions that connect places that are divided by water, roads, or a long drop. Bridge pose prepares the body for both Bow pose and Candle pose, so it is a good warm-up to both. See what type of bridge you make.

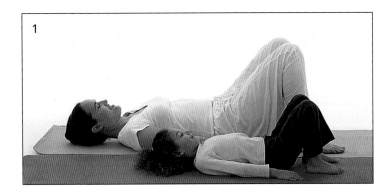

1 Lie on your back on your mat. Bend your knees and place your feet on the floor close to your bottom, a hip-width apart. Place your arms by your sides with your palms facing the floor.
Inhale: press your feet and palms into the floor and lift your pelvis.

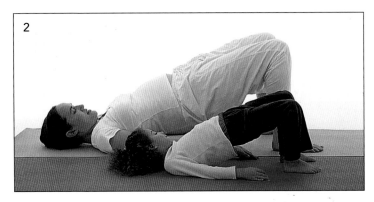

2 **Exhale:** start to raise your hips up as high as possible, supporting yourself on your shoulders and feet.

3 Keep pushing up until you are balancing on your shoulders and your feet and look like a bridge. Either interlace your hands behind your back or have them by your side to support your back. If this feels comfortable, then try the variation.

3

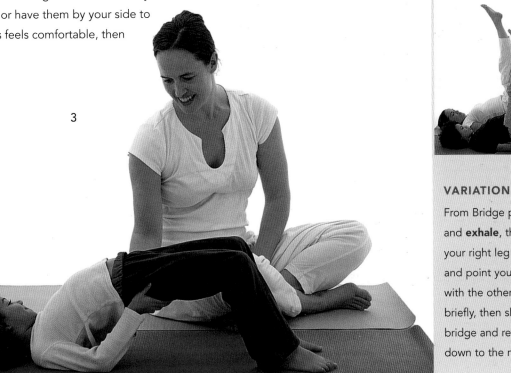

VARIATION

From Bridge pose, **inhale** and **exhale**, then extend your right leg straight up and point your toe. Repeat with the other leg. Hold briefly, then slowly lower the bridge and release back down to the mat.

Bow pose

Bow pose imitates a bow, as in a bow and arrow. Your arms become the string of the bow, creating tension between the upper body and the legs. It prepares you for more difficult back-bending poses, such as the Wheel. Find out how bendy you are.

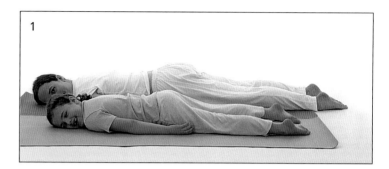

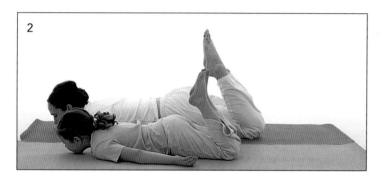

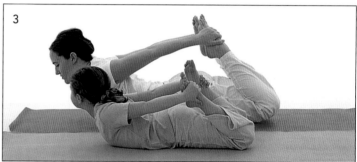

1 Lie on your mat on your tummy with your arms by your side. Place your head to the side.

2 **Inhale:** bend your knees toward your bottom.

3 Reach back and take hold of the tops of your feet with your hands.

Benefits

This pose massages the tummy, helping to improve digestion and getting rid of toxins. It keeps your spine supple, and can also relieve asthma symptoms.

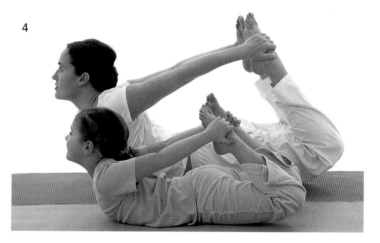

4 **Exhale:** lift your legs up and back. Keep your arms straight and allow the strength of your legs to lift up your chest. Look up, stretching out your neck. Hold briefly, then slowly release back down again.

5 To release all the tension in your back, crouch forward into Child's pose, tucking your legs in and keeping your arms by your sides.

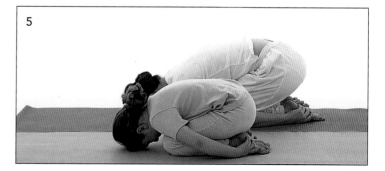

Wheel pose

Wheels are one of our greatest inventions. How would cars, trucks, or bicycles move without wheels? Enjoy making a large, round wheel. Learn this pose in a yoga class before practicing at home.

1 Lie on your back on your mat. Bend your knees and place your feet close to your bottom, about a hip-width apart.
Inhale: place your palms underneath your shoulders with your fingers pointing forward and your elbows straight up.

2 **Exhale:** press your palms and feet into the floor and raise up your hips. Let your head drop back and rest for a moment on the crown. Straighten your arms and legs and lift your belly as high as you can to make a tall bridge. Hold briefly, looking down toward the floor, and then slowly lower yourself back down again, tucking your chin in toward your chest. Now go into Child's pose (see Step 5 opposite) to ease your back.

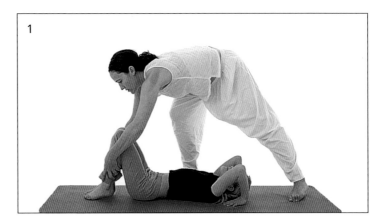

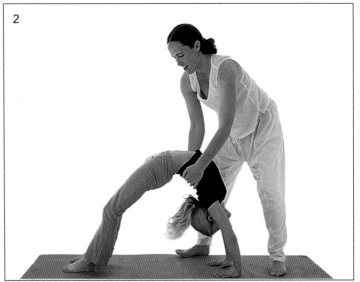

CHILD'S TIP
Help your child into the final position, as it is difficult to achieve.

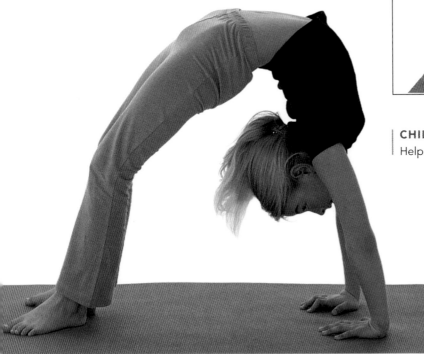

Benefits

This pose flexes and strengthens the spine. It stimulates and boosts the nervous system and the endocrine system.

Child's pose

This pose imitates the position of a baby in the mother's womb. It is a quiet, restful pose and can be done whenever you feel tired during a yoga class.

Kneel on your mat. Bend forward, rest your forehead on the floor, and rest your arms by your body.
Breath: breathe deeply and completely relax. Hold the pose for as long as it is comfortable, then slowly come up.

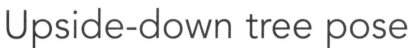

Benefits
This pose relaxes the mind and relieves any tension in the back.

Upside-down tree pose

A good way to turn your world around and look at it from a new angle is to become an upside-down tree. To do this handstand you need to balance well.

Start standing close to a wall, or have an adult to help you.
Inhale: bend forward and place your hands, with your fingers spread, on the floor close to the wall.
Exhale: kick your legs up against the wall (or get an adult to help and hold you), so that you are completely inverted. Rest your feet against the wall, or balance on your own. Hold briefly, then come down and rest in Child's pose (see above).

Benefits
Upside-down tree pose strengthens the wrists and arms and clears your mind by sending fresh blood rushing to your brain.

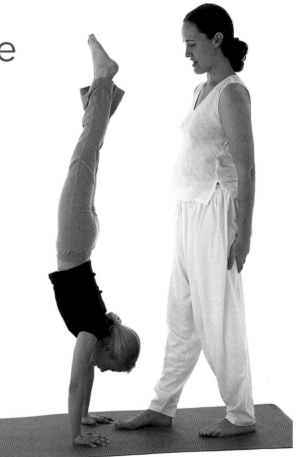

Candle pose

Light up the world with this pose! Candle pose is also known as a shoulder stand, and it is an easy pose for you to do. Learn this pose in a yoga class before practicing at home.

1 Lie on your back on your mat with your legs together and arms close to your body, with your palms facing down.

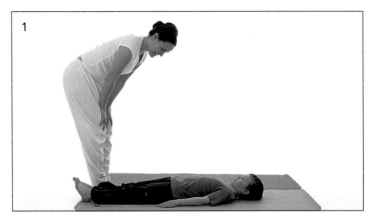

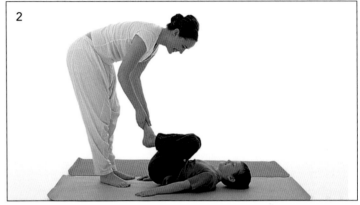

2 Inhale: bend your knees toward your chest and slowly start to swing them over your head.

3 Exhale: straighten your legs and support your back with your hands. Stretch your legs straight up and feel your body weight evenly distributed between your elbows, your shoulders, and the back of your head. Hold this pose for 10–20 seconds. To come down, bend your knees toward your forehead, place your hands on the floor, palms down, and slowly roll out of the pose, one vertebra at a time.

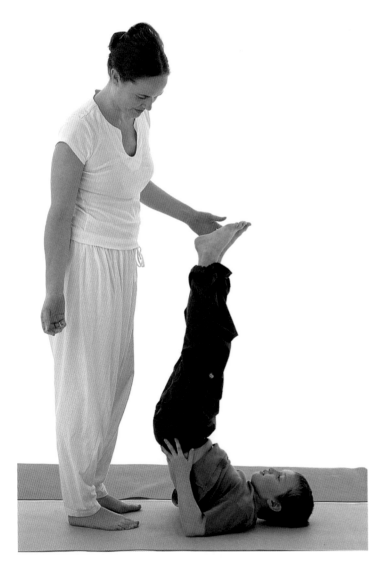

PARENT'S TIP

Your child may need some support in this pose. It has a powerful effect on the thyroid and parathyroid glands, so only let him or her hold the pose for short periods. If a child has neck or back injuries, this pose and Plow pose (see page 77) should be avoided.

Candle pose using a wall

If you are finding Candle pose difficult, practice using a wall for support.

1 Place the end of your yoga mat against a wall. Lie on one side with both knees bent and place your buttocks close to the wall. **Inhale:** roll to the side and extend both your legs up the wall. Place your buttocks as close to the wall as possible and make sure that your torso and head are in a straight line.

2 Bend both your knees and place the soles of your feet on the wall.

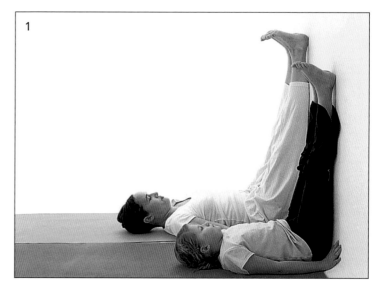

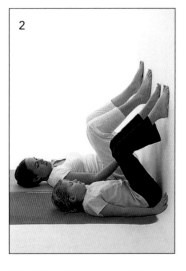

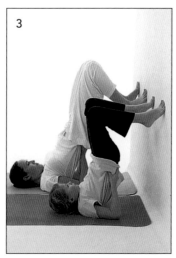

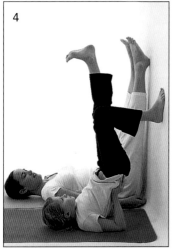

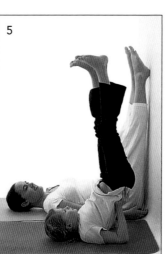

3 **Exhale:** press your feet against the wall and lift your hips and back off the floor. Bend your elbows and support your back with both hands. Press your pelvis forward to form a straight line from the shoulders to the knees.

4 **Inhale, exhale,** and when balanced, slowly raise one leg straight up in the air.

5 Now raise the other leg up into Candle pose. Hold briefly, then bend your knees and place the soles of your feet on the wall, then gently release your buttocks to the floor.

Plow pose

Plow pose is a natural extension of Candle pose, and sends fresh blood to your brain, giving you lots of new thoughts and ideas. Learn this pose in a yoga class before practicing at home.

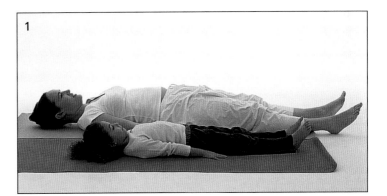

1 Lie on your back on your mat with your legs together and arms close to your body with your palms facing down.

2 **Inhale:** lift up your legs and, keeping them straight, swing them over your head toward the floor.

Benefits

Plow pose regulates the hormones in the adrenal system, and also boosts the pancreas.

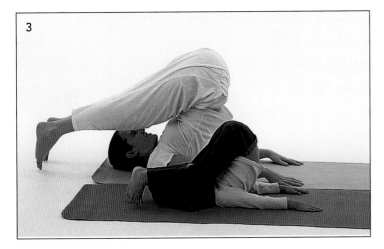

3 **Exhale:** as your feet touch the floor, stretch your arms away from your feet. To come out of the pose, place your palms on the floor and slowly roll out.

CHILD'S TIP
Be careful not to turn your head to the side in this pose; always keep it in the center.

Lotus pose

In India, a lotus flower represents increased knowledge and understanding. Imagine you are a beautiful lotus when in this position. Learn this pose in a yoga class before practicing at home.

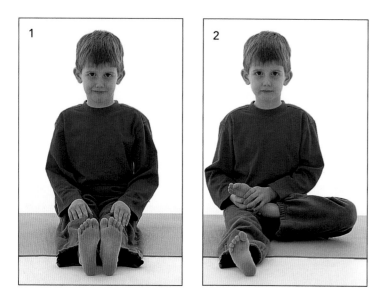

3

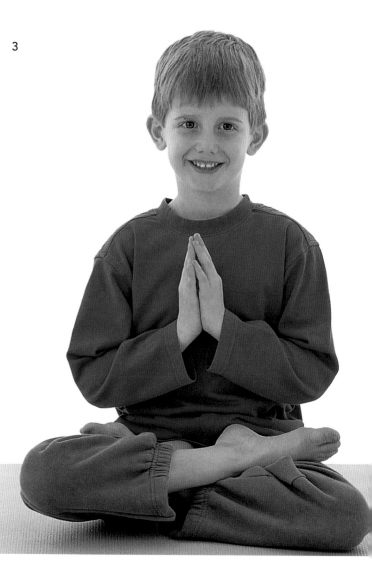

1 Sit on your mat with your feet straight out in front of you.

2 Bend your left leg and place your foot on top of your right thigh, with the sole facing upward.

3 If this feels comfortable, then bend your right leg, lift the foot, and place it on top of your left thigh. Keep your spine straight, relax your face and sit quietly for a few moments.

PARENT'S TIP
If a child has knee injuries, do not let them do this pose.

Jackknife pose

In this pose you learn how to fold completely in half, rotating from the hip joints, just like a jackknife.

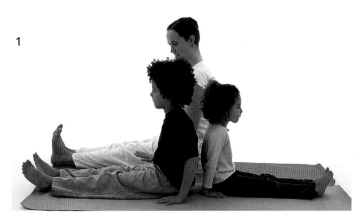

1 Sit upright on your mat with both your legs outstretched. Place the palms of your hands on the floor beside your hips and sit up tall, stretching your spine.

2 **Inhale:** stretch your arms up over your head, pulling up from the sit-bones (in your buttocks) to your fingertips.

3 **Exhale:** bend forward with a flat back over your straight legs and take hold of your toes, or as far down your legs as you can comfortably reach. Look toward your feet and keep extending your spine over your straight legs.
Breath: rest in this pose for a few breaths, then **inhale** and come up.

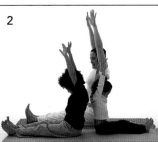

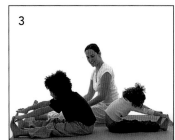

Benefits
Jackknife pose really stretches your back, calms your heart, and helps you digest your food.

Corkscrew pose

In this pose, imagine that your spine is like a corkscrew and see how far you can twist around.

1 Sit upright on your mat with both legs outstretched. Bend your right leg and place your foot on the mat on the outside of your left knee.
Inhale: lift up your spine and begin to twist toward your right leg, placing your right hand on the floor behind you.
Exhale: hook your upper arm on the outside of your right knee and use it as lever to move deeper into the twist. With your shoulders relaxed, twist up from the base of your spine, turning your hips, waist, chest, and shoulders. Now turn your head to look over your right shoulder. Hold briefly, then **inhale**, and turn back to center.

2 Repeat the twist on the other side to balance the stretch, hooking your arm on the outside of your left knee.

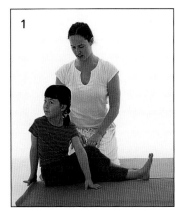

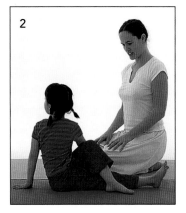

Benefits
This pose makes your spine more flexible and massages your tummy organs.

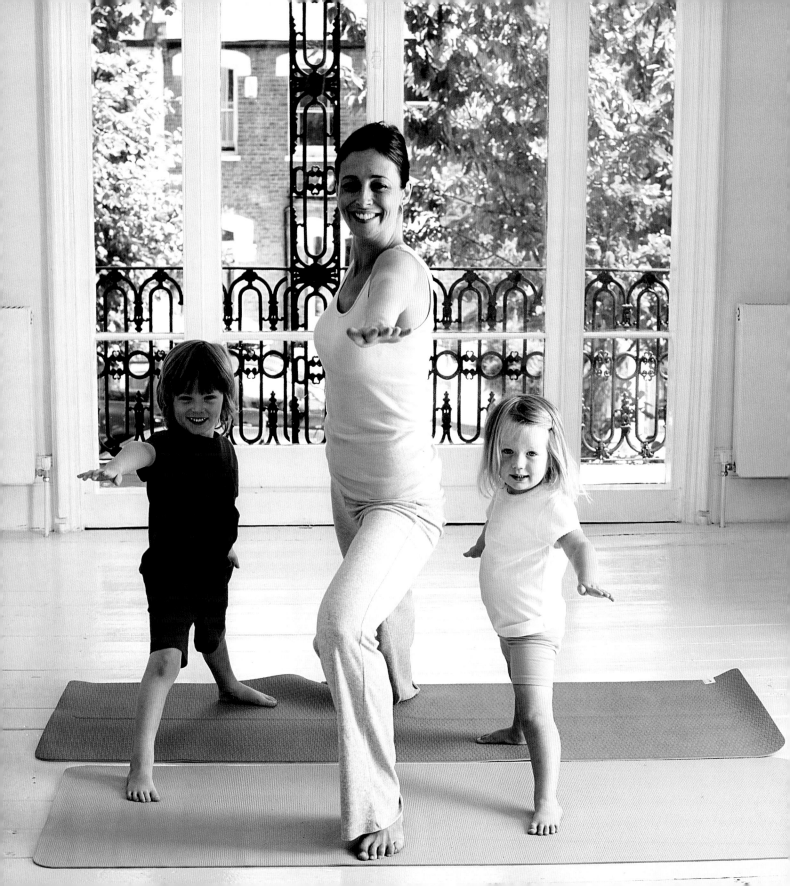

Chapter 5

Dynamic Poses

This series of lively postures moves smoothly from one pose to the next. Dynamic poses are energizing and especially good for older children (aged 7–11) to keep them interested and motivated. The poses create heat, so they promote flexibility in the body and use up excess energy. Practicing them regularly helps eliminate toxins, tones the muscles, strengthens the lungs, and boosts the digestive process. Practicing the poses with your children can give them extra confidence in attempting all the different movements.

Salute to the sun

The sun is by far the largest and brightest object in the solar system. Without the sun there would be no life on earth. Salute to the sun is a great energizer—stretching out the whole body—and is a great way to start a session. Generally, breathe in as you stretch upward and backward and out when you bend forward.

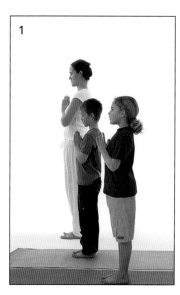

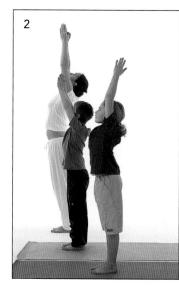

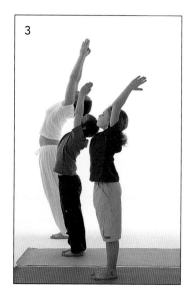

1 Stand upright in Mountain pose (see page 62) on your mat with your feet together and your hands together in Prayer pose.

2 Stretch your arms up above your head. Keep them a shoulder-width apart.

3 Lift up your chest and bend gently back, but do not strain your lower back.

4 Bend forward from your hips, keeping your back and knees straight. Relax your head down toward your knees and place your hands in line with your feet. If your hands do not touch the floor, bend your knees so they do.

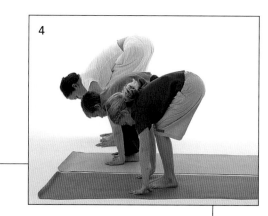

5 Stretch your left leg back and drop your left knee to the floor. Arch your back, lift your chest, and look up.

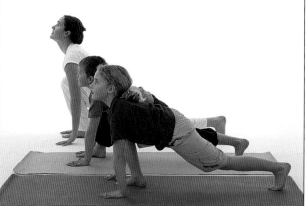

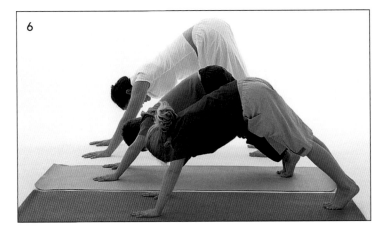

6

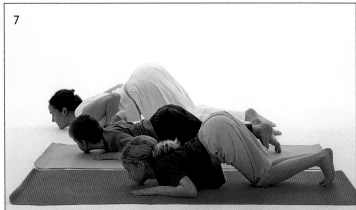

7

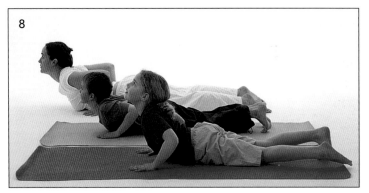

8

6 Now take your right foot back in line with your left foot, a hip-width apart. Go into Dog pose by pushing into your palms and lifting your buttocks up and back. Relax the back of your neck and look back between your feet. Press your heels down toward the floor.

7 Bend your knees to the floor and lower your chest to the floor between your hands, leaving your pelvis slightly raised. Place your chin on the floor.

8 Slide your body forward into Cobra pose (see page 53). Press into your palms, stretch out, and arch your spine. Lift up your chest and look up, but keep your pelvis on the floor.

9 Push into your hands, and raise your buttocks up and back, coming back into Dog pose, so that your body forms a triangle.

Relax the crown of your head toward the floor. Keep lengthening your spine and take your heels to the floor.

10 Step your right foot forward and bend your knee so that it lines up with your hands, and release your pelvis down. Lift your chest forward, lengthen your spine, and look up.

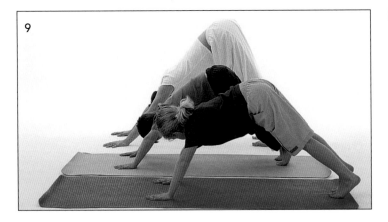

9

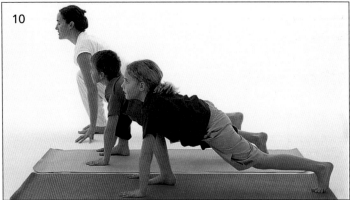

10

11 Bring your left foot forward in line with your right foot. Relax your head toward your knees and come into a forward bend.

12 Slowly come up, stretching your arms up close to your ears; then take them back, keeping your body in one straight line from your hips to your fingertips. Lift and open your chest and gently bend back.

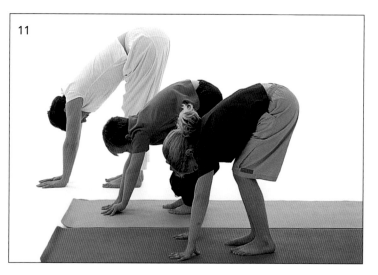

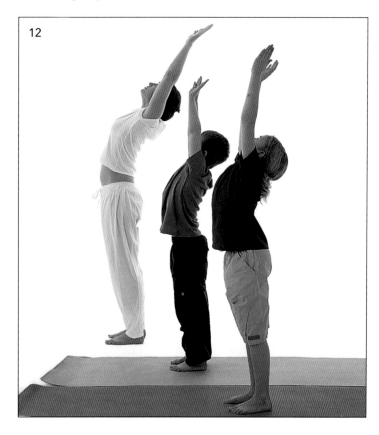

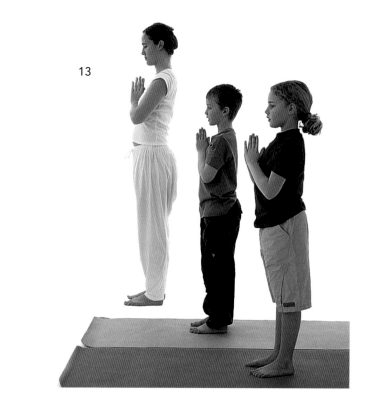

13 Bring your hands back down in Prayer position in front of your chest. Rest for a moment and then repeat the cycle, taking your right leg back first to complete one full round of Salute to the sun.

Benefits

Salute to the sun can improve coordination for growing children and help their concentration. The sequence increases the energy flow to all the muscles, joints, and major internal organs.

Salute to the moon 1

The moon is the second brightest object in the sky after the sun, although it does not radiate its own light, but reflects the sun. The gravitational pull between the earth and the moon creates tidal flow. This lively sequence helps to increase flexibility. Generally, breathe in as you stretch upward and backward and out when you bend forward.

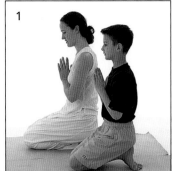

1 Start the pose sitting back on your heels on your mat, with your hands together in prayer position—*namaste*.

2 Go down onto all fours; keep your back straight, and try to keep your arms directly in line with your shoulders.

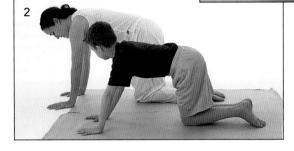

3 Step your left foot forward, between your hands. Start to lift your chest and look up.

4 With your weight on your left leg, bend backward, opening your chest and, lifting your arms up above your head, look upward. Hold briefly, then release.

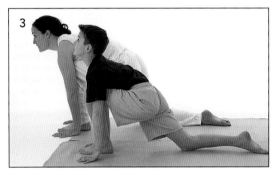

5 As you bring your arms down, go into Child's pose. Move into a kneeling position, then lean forward, tucking your head in with your arms at your side and resting on your heels like a tortoise to relax any tension in your spine.

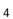

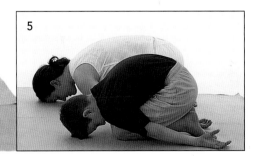

Salute to the moon 2

This variation on Salute to the moon 1 works on strengthening the muscles around the waist and the lower back.

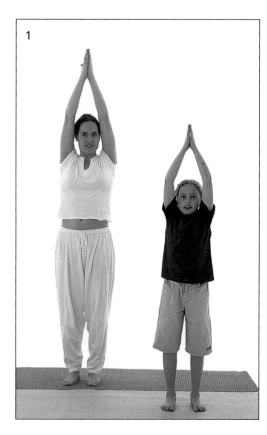

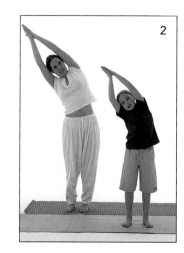

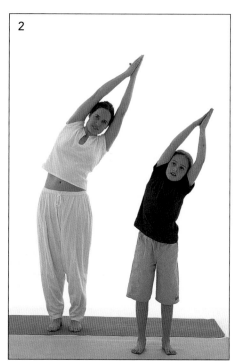

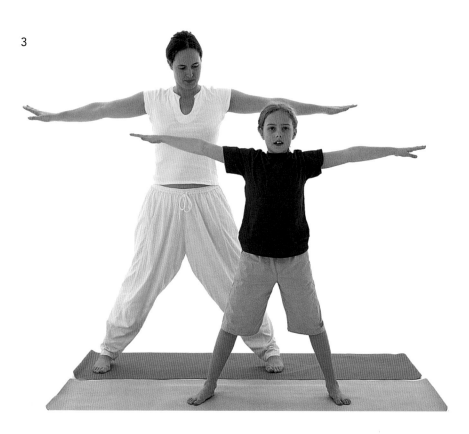

1 Stand upright in Mountain pose (see page 62) with your feet together and your palms together in prayer position—*namaste*. Lift your arms straight up above your head, and put your palms together.

2 Lean your body to the right for a few moments, and then to the left briefly as in Swaying palm tree pose (see page 63).

3 Release your hands. Jump your feet 3 ft/1 m apart, with your arms out at shoulder height.

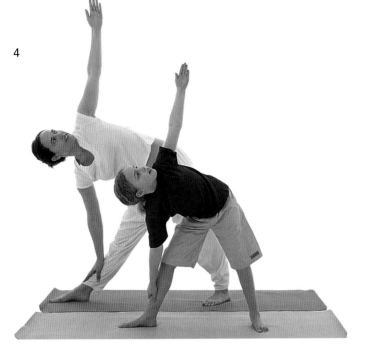

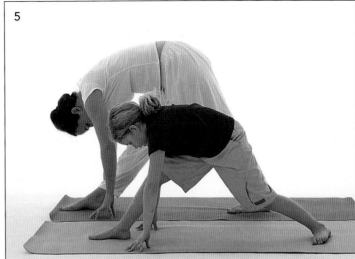

4 Turn your right foot out to point forward and keep your your left foot turned in slightly. Keeping your arms straight, extend your torso to the right and place your right hand on your right leg between the ankle and the thigh. Extend your left hand straight up, as in Triangle pose (see page 64).

5 Turn your hips and torso toward your right leg. Lower both hands toward your right foot and place them on the floor, then bend your head toward your right knee.

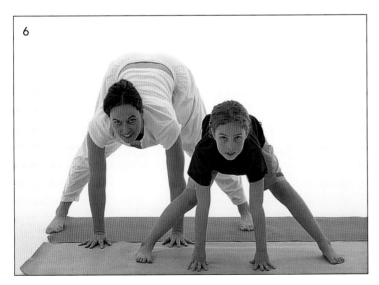

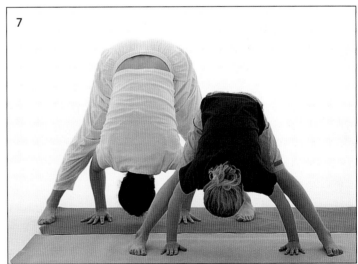

6 Walk your hands and turn your torso toward the front, placing your hands between your feet a shoulder-width apart. Turn your feet to the front.

7 Lower the crown of your head toward the floor, then work back to Step 5, bringing your left forward, come back up to standing, then rest.

Warrior pose

Warriors are strong and powerful. Some, like Spiderman, have superhuman strength, so boys particularly will enjoy this sequence.

1 Stand upright in Mountain pose (see page 62) with your palms together in prayer pose—*namaste*.

2 Extend your arms out to the sides and raise them above your head, back into Prayer position with palms together. Look up at your hands.

3 Bend forward from your hips, keeping your back and knees straight. Relax your head down toward your knees and place your hands in line with your feet. If your hands do not touch the floor, then bend your knees.

4 Step your left leg backward, ready for Downward dog pose (see page 44).

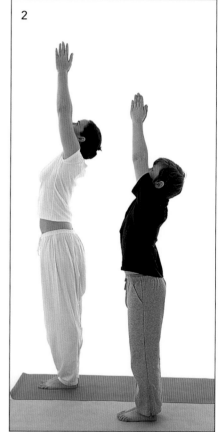

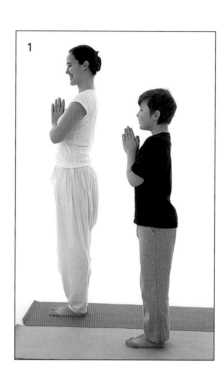

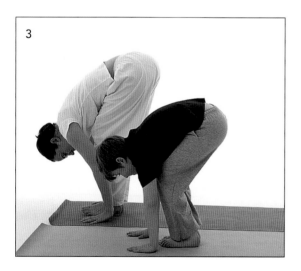

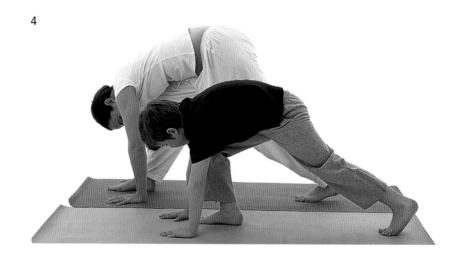

6

Warrior has some powerful moves; it builds strength, stamina, and gives you a fighter's confidence. It strengthens your legs, hips, back, and heart.

5

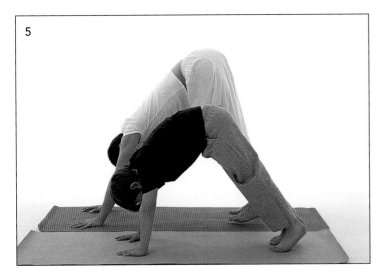

7

5 Step your right leg back, stretch your arms, and lift your tailbone right up into the air in Downward dog pose, hold for a few moments.

6 Step your right foot forward between your hands. While keeping your right knee bent, raise your torso and lift your arms over your head. Make sure they are a shoulder-width apart, with palms facing each other and straight elbows. Look up between your hands and hold briefly.

7 Turn your torso forward and extend your arms out at shoulder height. Keep your knee bent and look over your right shoulder. Then place your hands on the floor on either side of your bent leg and repeat the sequence from Step 4 with your left leg. Then follow Steps 3, 2 and finish with Step 1, with your hands back in Prayer position.

Row the boat pose

This pose can be fun to do in pairs so you can compare how well you are rowing the boat.

1 Sit up straight on your mat with your legs straight out in front. With your hands by your sides, imagine that you are about to start rowing a boat.

2 **Inhale:** raise your hands up over your head, stretching up from your chest.

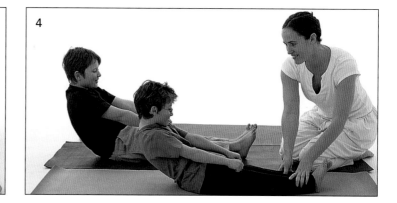

PARENT'S TIP
For more fun, you can get the children to try it in a group, with the next child sitting in front of the first, between their legs.

3 **Exhale:** bend forward, extending your hands toward your feet in a circular motion.

4 Slide your hands up your legs and lean back as far as you can without falling. Repeat Steps 1 and 2 (**inhaling** as you stretch up) in forward rowing movements 10 times, and then in reverse rowing movements 10 times.

Benefits
Rowing the boat pose strengthens your abdomen and flexes your hips.

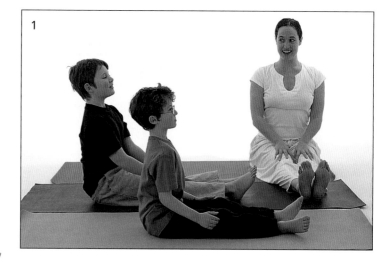

Bicycle pose

1 Lie on your back on the mat with your arms close to your body and palms facing down.

2 Raise your legs, so that they are perpendicular. Cycle your legs in mid-air as if you are riding a bike. Feel how forcefully your legs are doing the cycling movement, then lower your feet toward the floor until your heels are just off the floor. Reverse the movement and repeat Steps 1 and 2. Keep breathing evenly throughout.

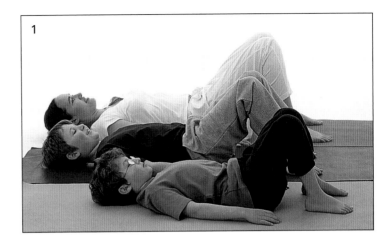

1

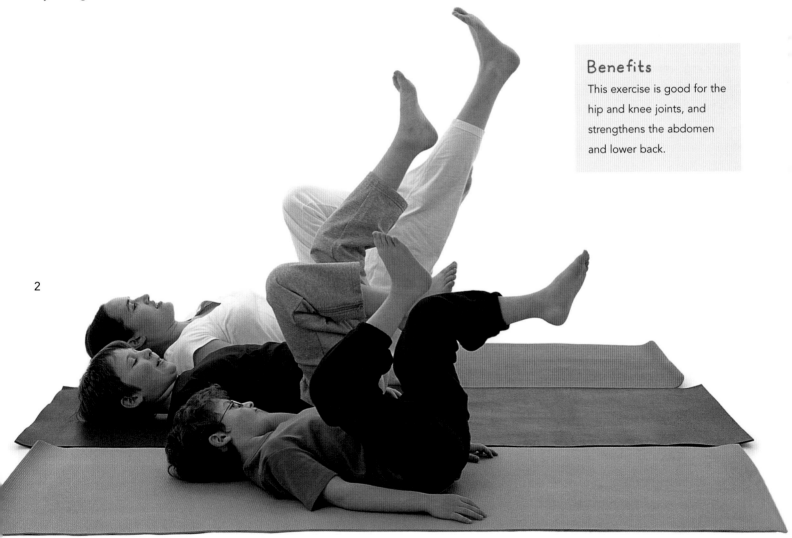

2

Benefits

This exercise is good for the hip and knee joints, and strengthens the abdomen and lower back.

Rock and roll pose

Both this exercise and Rolling splits (opposite) massage the entire spine as you roll along it. Be sure to do this exercise on a soft surface such as a folded blanket and keep your head tucked right in.

(opposite)

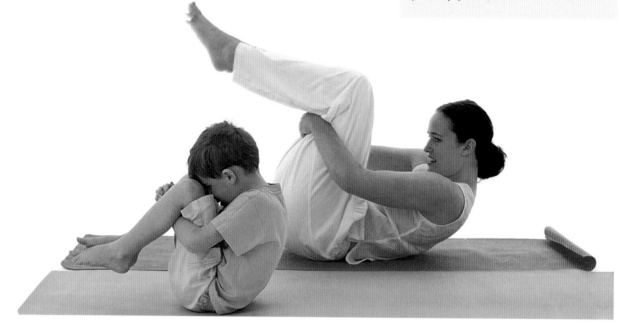

Benefits

This exercise massages your spine and perks up your mind.

1

1 Sit on your mat with your legs straight out in front of you. Bend your knees in toward your chest and clasp your hands under your knees. Tuck your chin in and lower your forehead toward your knees. Curl up your spine so that you are like a ball.

2 Slowly roll backward and forward along your spine. See if you can propel yourself with the movement of your legs. Keep breathing evenly throughout. Repeat 5–10 times.

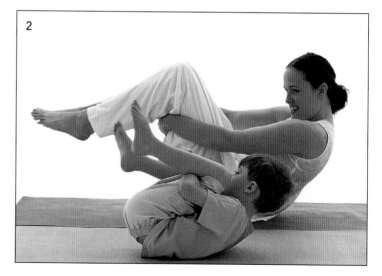

2

Rolling splits pose

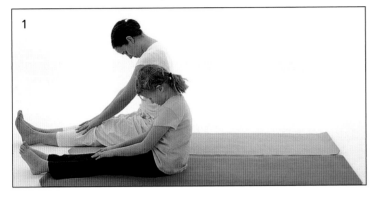

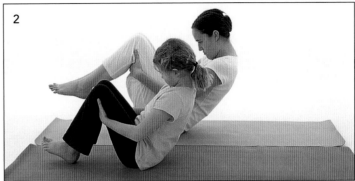

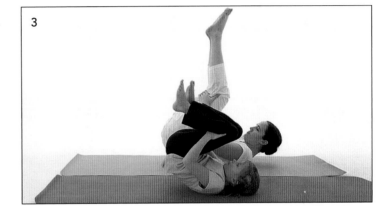

1 Start sitting on your mat with your legs straight out in front of you.

2 Bend your knees toward your chest and hold the backs of your knees. Curve your spine and tuck your chin in toward your chest.

3 Start to roll backward into Plow pose (see page 77), propelling yourself backward.

4 As you get into Plow pose, touch your feet on the floor behind your head.

5 Roll all the way forward until the backs of your legs touch the floor. Once sitting, bend forward toward the floor. Keep breathing evenly throughout. Repeat 5–10 times.

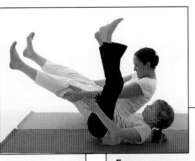

Benefits

This exercise stretches out your spine and increases flexibility in your hips.

Dynamic sit-up pose

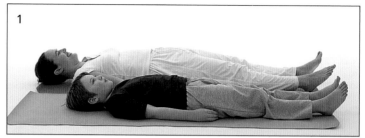

1 Lie flat on your back on your mat with your arms close to your body, palms facing down. Bring your legs together and flex your feet.

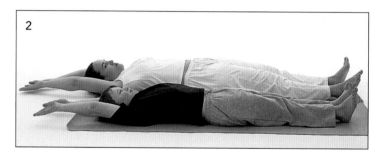

2 Stretch your arms over your head along the floor and then **inhale** deeply.

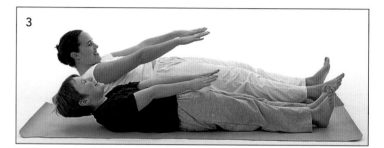

3 **Exhale:** lift up to a sitting position, keeping your tummy pulled in, then start to bend forward over your legs.

4 Reach toward your feet and stretch out your spine. Sit back up, extending your arms out in front, and slowly roll down to a lying position. Repeat from 5–10 times.

4

Benefits
This exercise strengthens your abdomen and lower back, and improves circulation, giving you more energy.

Striking cobra pose

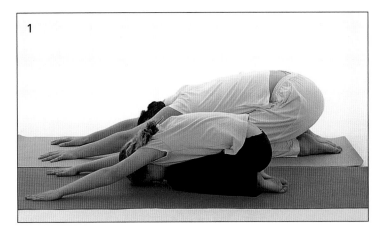

1 Come into Child's pose (see page 74), crouching on the mat with your arms extended out in front of you, palms facing down.

2 Move your chest forward, sliding it just above the floor until it is in line with your hands.

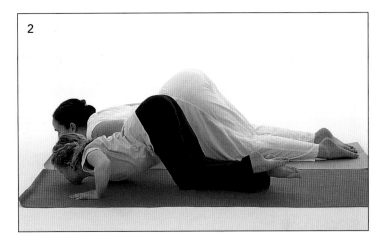

3 Lift your chest, arch your back, and straighten your arms. Lower your pelvis down to the floor, then look up and "hiss" loudly like a snake. Slowly raise your buttocks, bend your knees, and push backward into Child's pose once more. Repeat about 5–10 times.

CHILD'S TIP
Really enjoy hissing when you are in Step 3 and imagine you are a cobra.

Benefits

This exercise makes your spine more bendy and flexible. It also boosts the liver, kidneys, and intestines.

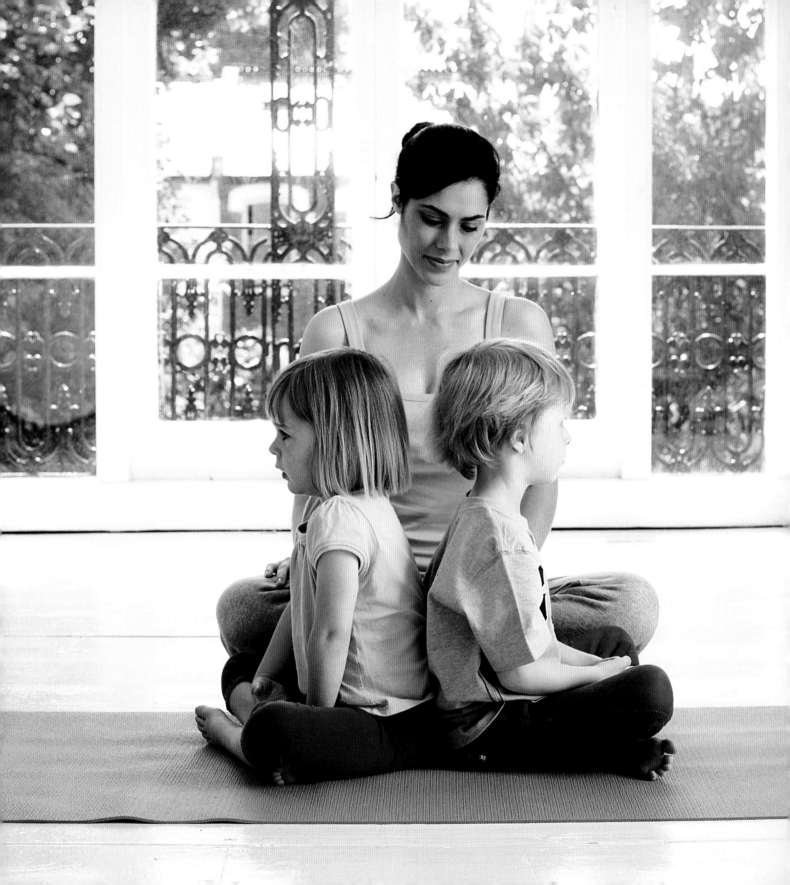

Chapter 6
Group Poses

Practicing yoga in a group or with a partner is a fun way to learn the yoga poses and to bond and interact with others. Children like working together. They will enjoy doing the poses as part of a group. In this chapter children can support and help each other to do the different poses. Partner yoga reduces the tendency for children to compete, and allows them to have fun with each other, improve their movements, and share their accomplishments with all their friends.

Blossoming lotus pose

The pose imitates the gentle unfolding of a flower. Be aware of the other children's movements, so that you can coordinate well with the rest of the group.

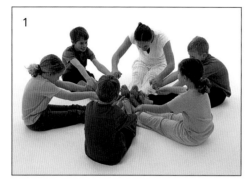

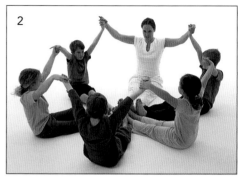

1 Sit in a circle on the floor with straight backs and holding hands. Point your feet toward the center. Coordinating your movements, bend forward and reach with your arms toward the center of the circle.

2 Slowly sit up and lift your arms in the air, stretching up from the waist.

3 Now start to lower your backs down toward the floor to lie down, bringing your arms out to the side.

PARENT'S TIP
To practice Blossoming lotus you need five or more kids.

4 Lie flat on the floor, making a beautiful lotus. Now lift up your right leg up and then your left leg. Slowly lower your legs and come back up to a sitting position. **Breath:** keep breathing evenly throughout. Repeat 3–5 times.

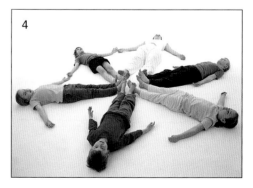

Wheelbarrow pose

Do this pose in pairs, and see how well you can move your partner around; or even race with your fellow wheelbarrows.

If you are going to be the wheelbarrow, come into Cobra pose (see page 53) on your mat. Let your partner gently lift up your legs, so that that you are balancing on your arms. Let your partner walk you backward and forward, and then change positions.

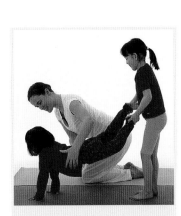

Benefits
This pose strengthens your arms and helps to make your shoulders more flexible.

King dancer

King dancer is a difficult balancing pose that becomes much easier with the help of a partner. Try and attempt the pose with your partner as a mirror image.

Make sure your partner is about the same height. Stand opposite each other, about 3 ft/1 m apart on your mat.
Inhale: both raise your left arms. Now, in unison, bend your right leg and take hold of your ankle.
Exhale: slowly kick your bent leg up and back as in Bow pose (see page 72) and tilt both your bodies forward, while supporting each other with your hands as you balance. Hold for a few moments, then release the leg down and repeat the pose on the opposite side.

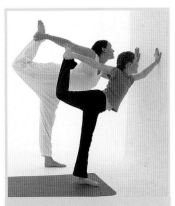

If you want to practice this pose on your own, use a wall for support as you balance.

Benefits
This pose strengthens your leg muscles and improves your balance and coordination.

Twists

Twisting is a great way to relieve any tense areas in your spine, and is even more fun when you do it with a partner who helps you to twist deeper.

1 Sit opposite each other with crossed legs on your mat.
Inhale: put your left arm behind your back and get your partner to do the same; twist slightly to the left.

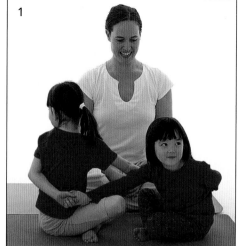

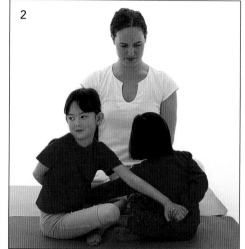

2 Exhale: take hold of your partner's right hand with your left, and hold their left hand with your right, and gently pull to twist more deeply. Feel the twist right from your spine up your shoulders.

Inhale: sit up and lengthen your spine.
Exhale: twist a little more. Hold briefly, then gently unwind. Repeat on the opposite side.

Boat pose with a partner

Boats float on water and carry people and cargo across the oceans. Practice this pose in twos or threes.

1 Sit on the floor on your mat opposite your partner with your knees bent, your toes touching, and holding hands.

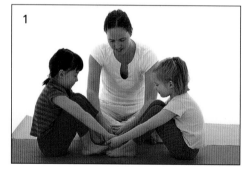

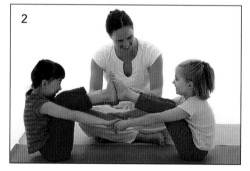

2 Inhale: lean slightly back, until your feet lift off the floor and you are balancing on your sit-bones (in your buttocks).

3 Exhale: touch the soles of your feet together and straighten your legs. Sing the song, "Row, row, row, your boat" together. Hold briefly, then release.

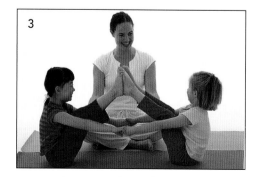

Benefits
Boat pose strengthens your tummy, back, and shoulder muscles. It also promotes good digestion.

Seesaw pose (back to back)

This pose is a fun way to practice forward bends with the help of a partner.

1 Sit in a cross-legged position on your mat with your back touching your partner's.
Inhale: place your hands on your knees and sit up very tall.

2 **Exhale:** slowly lean backward, gently pushing your partner forward as far as it is comfortable to go. Hold for a few seconds, then slowly sit upright again.

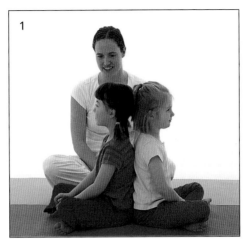

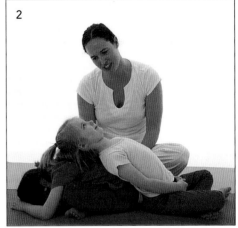

3 Repeat in the opposite direction with your partner leaning back so that you go forward. Hold for a few seconds, then slowly sit upright.

Benefits
This pose makes your hips and back more flexible.

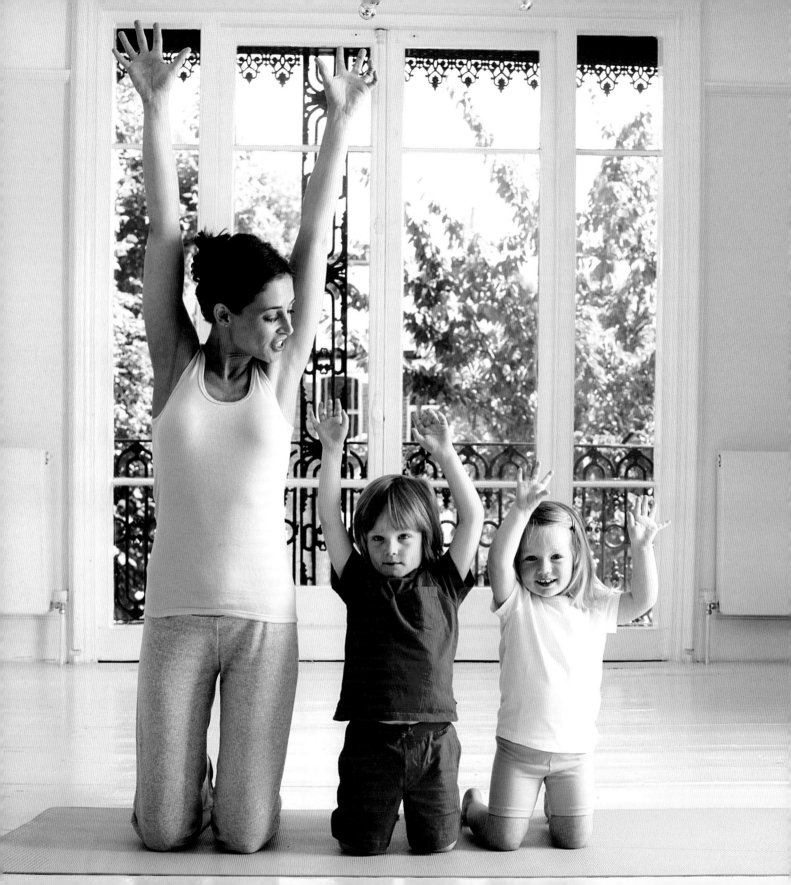

Chapter 7
Breathing

Breathing is essential to life. In yoga, it is believed that life and breath coexist. The air that we breathe keeps us alive, feeding our cells, tissues, nerves, glands, and organs. The amount of oxygen we take in influences all our bodily functions, from digestion to creative thinking.

This chapter contains some deep breathing exercises to teach children how to breathe fully from their diaphragms, opening up their chests, allowing their lungs to expand fully, improving their respiratory systems and massaging organs such as the heart and stomach. A well-balanced diet is also discussed as it is important to enable children to grow up strong and healthy.

Breathing

When we breathe in oxygen, it enters our lungs, where it is absorbed into the bloodstream. It then combines with glucose in the blood and produces energy. When we breathe out, carbon dioxide, a by-product of burning glucose, is released.

According to the yoga sutras, air contains *prana*, or vital life-force energy. We absorb *prana* through breathing, from sunshine, water, and food. When our bodies are filled with *prana*, our resistance to illness increases.

Breathing not only feeds the body, but how we breathe changes the way we think, as it has a direct effect on our minds and emotions. When our breathing is steady and deep, the mind is calmed and our nerves are soothed. Deep breathing gives the mind mental stability and sharpens the senses. The brain requires three times more oxygen than any other organ of the body to function efficiently.

Deep, rhythmic breathing is the quickest way to re-energize a tired body. Deep breathing also slows and relaxes the heart. The yoga texts say that our breath is linked to our natural rhythm. Each individual has a different rhythm and through the breath you are connected to your own rhythm, and equilibrium is established.

Most of us breathe too shallowly, particularly in times of stress, and stale air becomes trapped in the lungs, causing a build-up of toxins in the body.

Breathing and children

Breathing exercises are a great gift for children that can serve them throughout their lives. The different breathing exercises below can calm their nerves or increase energy. Showing your children how to breathe properly is also a great way to promote inner tranquility and build confidence. If you add in some visualization techniques with the breathing exercises, you can help increase their self-awareness and self-esteem. As they breathe in, teach them to imagine the qualities that they want to develop in themselves, such as strength, courage, self-confidence, or being good at a sport. As they exhale, let them breathe out all the unwanted aspects of their lives, such as unkind friends, illness, or not achieving at math or history.

Breathing exercises

You can perform most of the breathing exercises either sitting crossed-legged on your mat with a long spine or on your knees with your buttocks, resting on your heels, as a slouched posture can restrict how well you breathe. Make sure that the room is well ventilated and not too cold before you exercise.

Relaxed tummy breath

This simple exercise teaches you how to breathe completely, using your diaphragm. This requires less energy than breathing into the upper chest, and the exchange of oxygen and carbon dioxide is greater. Practice it either lying down or sitting up. If you are under the age of eight, it can be fun to practice the breathing lying down with a beanie toy, small boat, or favorite toy placed on your tummy, to focus your awareness.

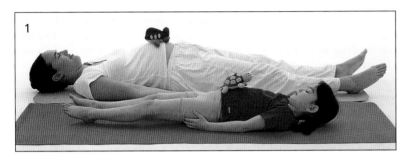

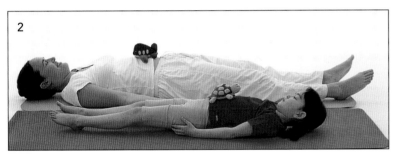

1 Lie down on your back on your mat. Place a small toy on your tummy near your navel.
Inhale: fill your belly with air so that your toy rises.

2 **Exhale:** draw your navel in toward your spine so that your toy sinks down again. You can imagine that the movement of your tummy is like the waves on the ocean.
Breath: continue breathing in and out for 10 breaths.

Blowing a fly off the end of the nose

Breathing rapidly from the diaphragm is very energizing. It helps to remove stale air and improve digestion.

Sit upright on your knees on your mat. Place your hand on your tummy. **Inhale** deeply through your nose, then **exhale** forcefully as you pull your tummy back toward your spine. As you do this, imagine that you are trying to blow a fly off the end of your nose with your breath. Repeat about 6–10 times.

Calming breath

This technique balances the left and right sides of your brain as cool air enters each nostril. With blocked nostrils, place your hands on your knees and imagine the air entering your nostrils: lifting your right index finger for right nostril and left index finger for your left nostril.

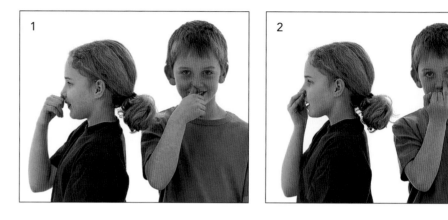

1 Sit upright on your knees on your mat. Bend your right arm and make a fist with the right hand. Release your thumb, ring and little fingers. Close your right nostril with your thumb.
Exhale, let out air through your left nostril.
Inhale, slowly and deeply, through the same nostril.

2 Let go with your thumb and, holding your left nostril with the ring finger, **exhale** through your right nostril.
Inhale through the same nostril and repeat the cycle 10 times.

Deep breathing

Yogic breath or deep breathing shows you how to use your lungs to their full capacity, which sends a flood of oxygen-rich blood through your body to stimulate your organs. Use either a feather or a plastic windmill for this exercise.

Inhale deeply, first filling your tummy with air, followed by your lower rib cage and then your upper lungs, until your chest and collar bones rise. When your lungs are completely full, **exhale** slowly, first from the top of your lungs, then the lower rib cage, and finally your tummy, moving your feather or windmill. Repeat a few times, then breathe normally again.

CHILD'S TIP
See how much you can move your feather or windmill as you practice this exercise.

A healthy diet

Eating a balanced diet with plenty of fresh fruit and vegetables gives the body the vital nutrients it needs to grow and thrive. By eating well, the body is cleansed, toxins are eliminated, and the vitamins and minerals that the body requires are easily absorbed. The aim of yoga is to lead a simple, healthy, and natural life. It is important to teach children at a young age how a good diet, ideally with small regular meals, encourages good health, energy, vitality, and a positive mental attitude. If they are encouraged to eat healthily from a young age, it will give them a firm foundation for the rest of their lives.

Yogic foods

In yoga, there is no perfect diet, and children's food requirements will depend on their constitution. In yoga philosophy, foods that are full of nutrients are called *sattvic*. This term refers to the type of energy contained in the food source. *Sattvic* foods are fresh ingredients that are not spicy, and include live yogurt, fruits, nuts, vegetables, cooked grains, and cereal. These foods increase energy and create balance in the body. Yogis advocate a vegetarian diet, as one of the basic principles of yoga is to not harm any living creature.

Foods that can make children hyperactive or restless are called *rajasic*. *Rajasic* foods include: sweets, tea, coffee, spices, meat, eggs, fish and food additives, and

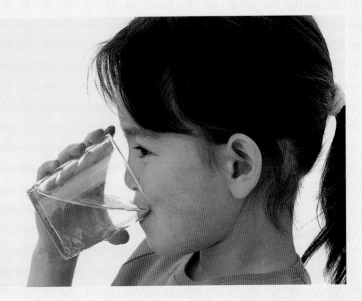

Drink a glass of water about every hour to keep your body hydrated.

colorings. These all have a stimulating effect on the body. Following the yoga principles, it is best to eat small amounts of these foods.

Foods that are over-cultivated, processed, stale, deep-fried, or refined are called *tamasic*. These foods are best avoided. They include fast foods, and can make your stomach feel heavy and encourage lethargy.

The benefits of water

Water is essential for survival—our bodies are made up of 70 percent water. It helps us to digest and eliminate our food. Ideally, we need about 4 pt/2 liters of water a day, half of which can be extracted from a diet high in fresh vegetables and salads. Drinking tea, coffee, and sugary drinks increases the need for water. Encourage children to drink still water rather than carbonated or sugary drinks, as it is the best way to cleanse the body and keep it healthy and functioning well.

Eat a piece of fresh fruit, rather than candies, to give your body plenty of nutrients.

Breath and movement

In yoga, all the exercise movements are done in unison with the way you breathe, generally expanding the diaphragm on an inhalation and contracting it on an exhalation. To learn how to coordinate your breath and movement, try practicing these simple exercises.

Sprouting seed

1 Start curled forward on your mat in Child's pose (see page 74) and imagine that you are a tiny seed in the ground.

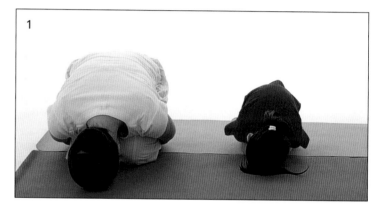

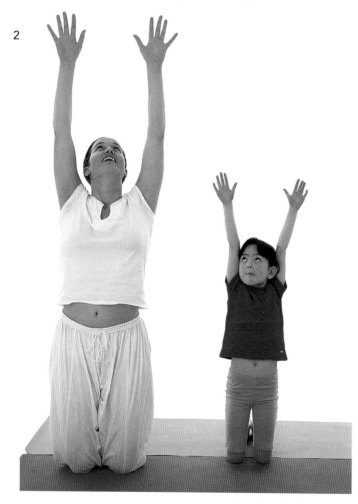

2 **Inhale:** imagine that you have started to grow. Lift up onto your knees and raise your arms above your head. On the full stretch, hold your breath for a moment.

Exhale: release your arms, and curl back down into a tiny seed. Repeat 3–6 times.

Huggy bear

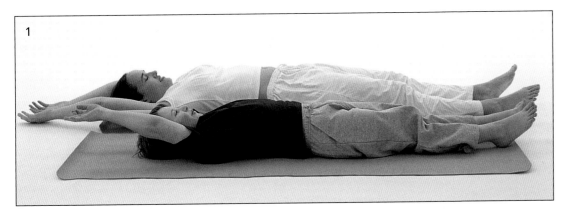

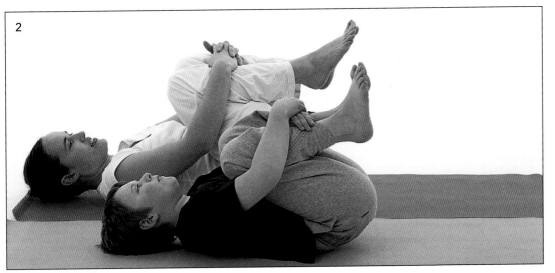

1 Lie flat on your back on your mat.
Inhale: raise your arms over your head.

2 **Exhale**, make a "Ha" sound, and hug your knees into your chest. Try not to lift your head, then release back onto the mat. Repeat 3–6 times.

BREATHING AND ASTHMA

Asthma in children is on the increase. The basic symptoms of asthma are the contraction of the tubes of the lungs and the over-production of mucus, which further obstructs the airways. An asthma attack results in excruciating breathlessness, especially when breathing out. The cause of asthma is a combination of many factors: pollution, diet, and stress. Children with asthma are often caught in a vicious cycle that compounds the problem. Yoga poses and breathing exercises, combined with conventional and alternative medicine, can help alleviate asthma symptoms.

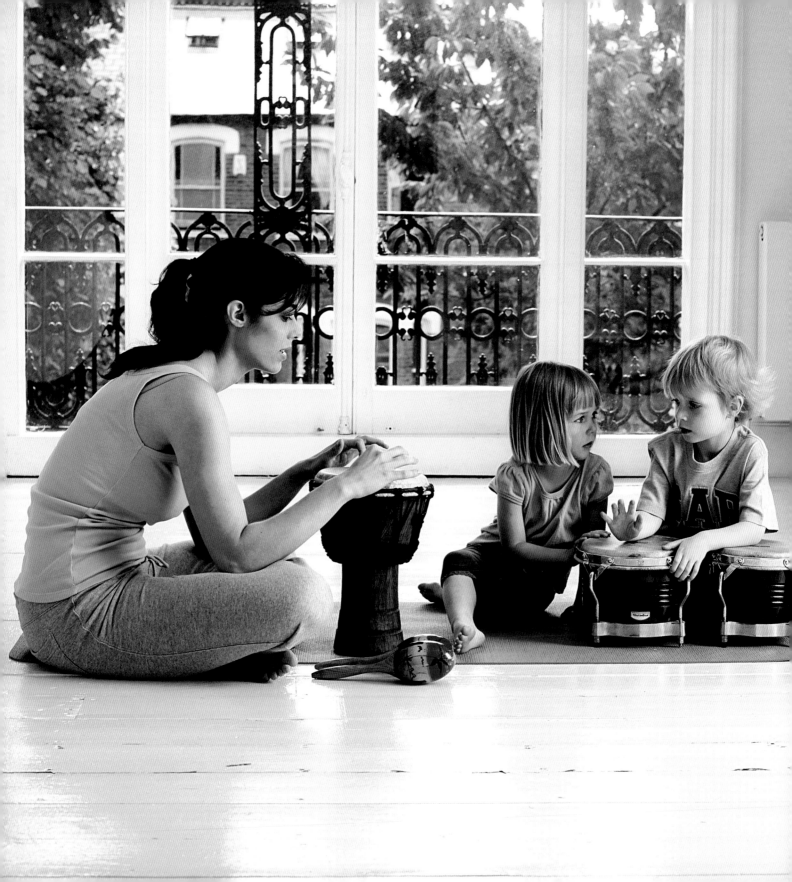

Chapter 8

Exploring the Senses

The mind is like the control tower of the body, receiving and sorting information and overseeing all physical activities. Being able to harness and control the constantly active mind is the goal of yoga.

This chapter contains simple exercises that work with the senses, and there is a section on relaxation at the end. Getting children to focus on a single object, such as a flower, can calm their minds and help them to cope better with any emotional ups and downs. When they practice listening to sounds, it improves their hearing and concentration, while chanting tones their vocal cords, and exercising their eyes can improve their vision.

Eyes around the clock

Sit in a comfortable seated position on your mat or on a chair. Imagine that you have a large clock face in front of you, or ask an adult to draw one for you to look at.

CHILD'S TIP
Rub the palms of your hands briskly together until they feel hot, and gently cup them over your eyes. The heat will relax your eye muscles.

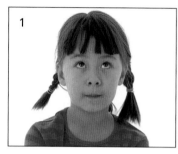

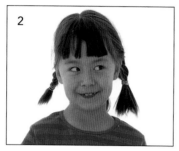

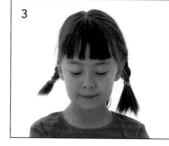

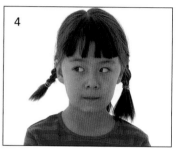

1 Start by moving your eyes up and down. Look up toward twelve o'clock.

2 Now move your eyes down in a straight line toward six o'clock. Repeat a few times, then close your eyes and rest.

3 Now move your eyes from side to side. Move your eyes to the right and look toward three o'clock.

4 Now move your eyes in a straight line toward nine o'clock on your left. Repeat 4–10 times, then close your eyes and rest. Finally, go around the whole clock. Take your eyes up to twelve o'clock and then to the right, looking at every number on the clock from one o'clock down to six o'clock.

Benefits
These eye exercises tone the optic nerves and improve peripheral vision.

Visualization with flower

PARENT'S TIP
Drawing the object from memory after studying it for a while helps children to become more observant and increases their awareness.

This exercise helps to balance and enhance the activities of the pineal gland, boosting intuition and helping to balance the emotions. Do this exercise on your own or in groups.

Sit on your mat. Place an object, such as a beautiful flower or shell, in front of you to look at. Stare at the object intently for 30 seconds. Now close your eyes and try to see the object in front of you in your mind. Repeat 4–10 times.

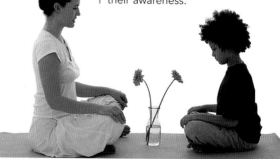

Chanting

This is a great way to focus young minds and release any pent-up energy. Children love to sing and make noise, and appreciate musical rhythm. Studies have shown that early exposure to music and rhythm not only increases musical ability but also improves a child's spatial awareness and ability to learn mathematics and logic.

Chanting strengthens the larynx, helping to develop communication skills, which makes the voice strong and expressive. It also energizes, creates a feeling of peace, and harmonizes a group of children chanting together.

Chanting differs from singing in that it repeats a few syllables, slightly varying the rhythm each round. It is fun to include some simple musical instruments such as tambourines or maracas, or the children can just clap in time to the rhythm.

See how good you feel when you start chanting. Singing or chanting exercises the vocal cords, and helps with releasing emotion. Do this exercise with some friends.

Different chants

The best-known Indian chant is the repetition of the sound, "OM," the sound is said to be the universal sound that embodies harmony and peace. The following is a list of simple Indian chants that can be used.

• *Om Shanti* means "OM peace."

• *Hari Om* is a healing mantra; *hari* is the divine sound for the Hindu deity Vishnu, who removes all impurities. The HA sound stimulates energy in the solar plexus, the RI sound moves the energy up to the throat, and the OM vibration is felt in the head.

• *Om namah Sivaya* is a chant to the deity Shiva, who destroys illusion and ignorance.

Alternatively, make up your own chants or use a line from a favorite nursery rhythm, such as "Twinkle, twinkle little star" and recite it repeatedly, or boost self-confidence by chanting positive affirmations such as "I am joy, I am peace."

Certain vowel sounds also activate different glands, so enhance children's communication skills by getting them to chant different vowel sounds or seed syllables while imagining the sound emanating from a different part of the body.

• Chant HA and feel the vibration in the solar plexus, stimulating the adrenals.

• Chant OU-O and experience the sound in the chest activating the thymus gland.

• Chant EA and feel the sound in the throat stimulating the thyroid and parathyroid glands.

• Chant EE and imagine the vibration between the eyebrows stimulating the pituitary gland.

• Chant AAH and feel the vibration in the head, helping to clear the brain, eyes, and nose.

Sit in a circle on a mat. Use some instruments such as a drum, tambourine, and rattle to create a musical rhythm. Then start chanting, choosing one from above, and see how good you feel as the chanting gets stronger. Notice where the sound is vibrating from. Practice the chanting for about 5–10 minutes.

Concentration with sound

Learn how to tune in to your environment by listening to some musical instruments. A tambourine and a rattle make different, distinctive sounds. Do this exercise on your own or in groups.

Sit on your mat on your own, or in a circle with other children. Close your eyes and listen carefully. When you hear the sound of the tambourine or rattle, open your eyes or put your hand up and say what you think it is.

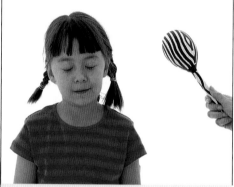

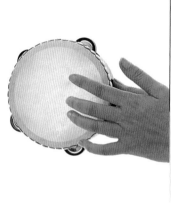

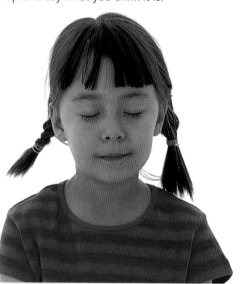

PARENT'S TIP

To increase the children's awareness of a space, make the sounds in different areas of the room and ask them to point to where they are coming from with their eyes closed. You can also get children to listen to the rustling of leaves or bird sounds.

Benefits
This exercise increases your sense of hearing, and its acuteness.

Relaxation

One of the most important yoga exercises for deep relaxation is Yoga *Nidra* or yogic sleep. You can practice yogic sleep by lying on your back and remaining completely still for 5–10 minutes. Lying quietly at the end of a yoga session allows the nervous system to assimilate all the benefits of the yoga poses. However, because relaxation is particularly difficult for children who are naturally full of energy, it is useful to practice yogic sleep at the beginning of a session, as well as at the end, to calm them down in preparation for a session.

Keeping warm

As all children's body temperatures will drop when they are lying down, it is a good idea to cover them with soft warm blankets or towels. Some children can feel vulnerable when they are lying on their backs, so wrap them tightly in the blanket or let them lie on their tummies instead. Play some quiet, soothing music to create the right atmosphere. Turn the lights low, burn some incense or aromatherapy oils, and make sure there will be no interruptions, from telephones or people walking through the space, for example.

Yogic sleep

Lie on your back on your mat. Place your feet a shoulder-width apart and drop them out to the sides. Place your arms a little way from your body and turn your hands, palms up. Slowly roll your head from side to side to release any tension in your neck. Completely release your body to the floor and breathe softly and gently. Go through your body, starting at your feet, tensing and relaxing each area. Now tighten all the muscles on your right leg, then let them go. Repeat with your left leg. Stretch out your arms and spread your fingers wide, then make fists with your hands. Tense all the muscles of your arms, and let them go. Take a deep breath in your tummy, filling it with air like a big balloon, then release the air through your open mouth with a loud "Ha" sound. Tighten all the muscles in your face toward the tip of your nose, and release. Finally, tighten your whole body, hold it for 5–10 seconds, and then completely relax like a floppy rag doll. Clear your mind of all thoughts and feel completely at peace. Stay awake, yet feel totally relaxed and calm.

Visualization exercises

Lead the children through this visualization exercise with a soft, soothing voice to help keep them awake.

Butterfly visualization

Imagine your body becoming very light. Now see yourself as a beautiful butterfly with bright, colorful wings sitting on a big, bright flower. Smell the flower, notice how it smells sweet, like vanilla. Feel a soft, warm gentle breeze against your wings as you flit amongst the flowers. See the big blue sky above you. Flap your wings and fly; feel yourself flying over trees, hills, and houses. You can fly wherever you want to go. Take the next few minutes to go wherever you wish. Now it is time to fly home. Imagine yourself landing on the same big bright flower. Take a nice big breath, and smell the flower.

PARENT'S TIP
A good way to end the relaxation session is by chanting the sound "OM" together to relax the mind further.

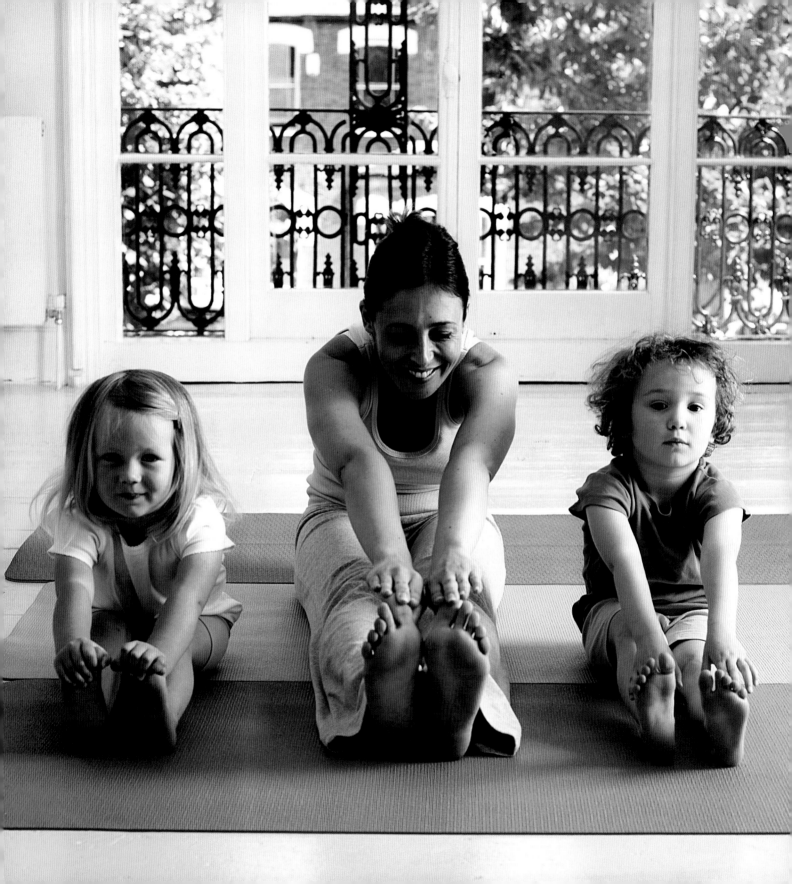

Chapter 9

Workouts

This chapter includes five yoga workouts: one is a short 20-minute workout for daily practice, or when you are short of time; the second one is for 3–6 year-old children to do with their parents; the third is for 7–11 year-old children to do with their parents; the fourth is an energizing workout (ideally for mornings) to boost tired children; and the fifth is a calming workout (ideally for afternoons) when children are stressed or overactive.

If your child cannot do a pose, then skip it and move on to the next. Aim to practice each pose twice, or as indicated.

Workouts

Traditionally in India, yoga poses are practiced every day except for Sundays or new moon and full moon days. Doing yoga every day cleanses your body internally and keeps it supple, strong, and healthy. It is better to practice yoga every day for 20 minutes than to do it occasionally for a longer period. However, with so many demands on parents' and children's time, it is difficult to commit to a daily routine, so try and practice together two to three times a week, and then you will really begin to appreciate the benefits of yoga.

The best times to practice

Try and do the poses early in the morning when your mind is fresh or sometime after school, to help all the family unwind. Do each pose once, or as indicated in the workout. Make sure that you practice in a quiet place, on an empty stomach, and wear some loose, comfortable clothing.

20-minute workout

This is an ideal workout for children to do daily, as it features warming-up exercises, a couple of standing poses, some sitting poses, and some relaxation exercises. If you only have ten minutes, practice the Salutation to the sun sequence (see pages 82–84) a few times.

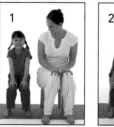

1 Yogic sleep (2–5 minutes) p.115

2 Jiggling p.32

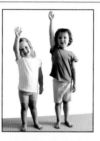

3 Windmill circles p.33

4 Shoulder shrugs p.35

5 Foot rotations p.36

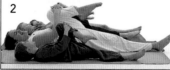

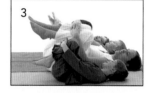

6 Knee to chest p.38

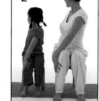
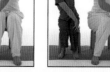

7 Sitting on a stool, side twist p.40

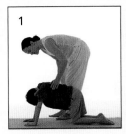

1

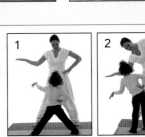

2

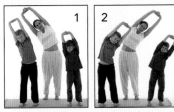

3

8 Cat pose p.45

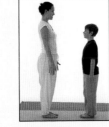

9 Mountain pose p. 62

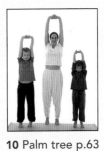

10 Palm tree p.63

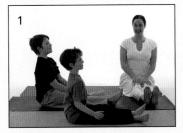

1   2

11 Swaying palm tree pose p.63

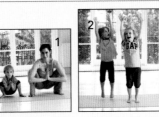

1   2

12 Teapot pose p.64

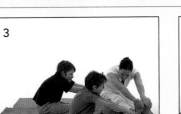

1   2

13 Frog pose p.51

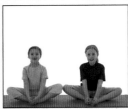

14 Butterfly pose p.57

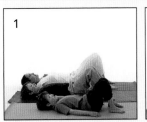

1

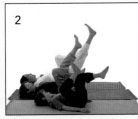

2

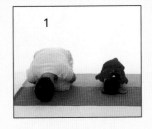

3

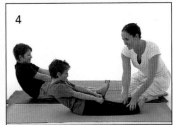

4

15 Row the boat pose p.90

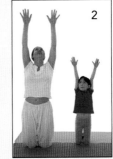

1   2

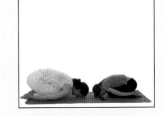

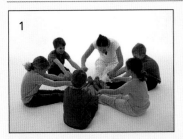

1

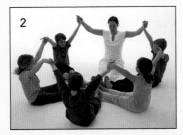

2

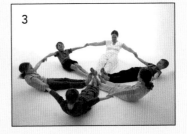

3

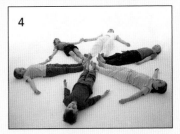

4

19 Blossoming lotus pose p.98

20 Yogic sleep p.115, see 1

Workout for 3–6 year-olds

45 mins

This fun workout includes some gentle breathing exercises and some Animal and Object poses. Try to make up a story out of the animals and objects used. During relaxation, teach your children simple anatomy by asking them to move different parts of their bodies.

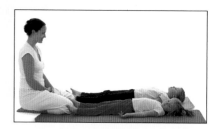

1 Yogic sleep (2–5 minutes) p.115

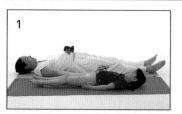

2 Relaxed tummy breath p.105

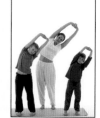

3 Huggy bear p.109

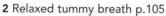

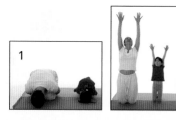

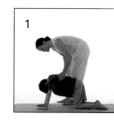

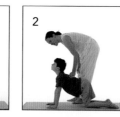

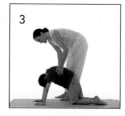

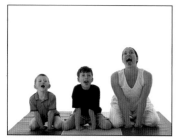

6 Lion pose p.46　**7** Mountain pose p.62　**8** Palm tree pose p.63　**9** Swaying palm tree pose p.63

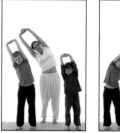

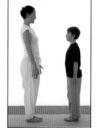

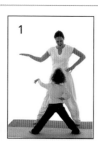

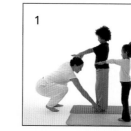

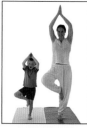

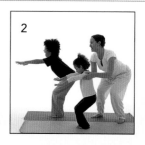

10 Tree pose p.62　**11** Teapot pose p.64　**12** Chair pose p.67

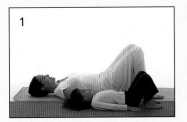
1

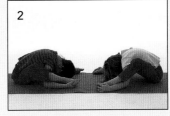
2

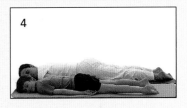
3

13 Bridge pose p.71

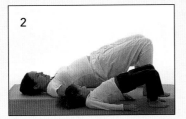
1

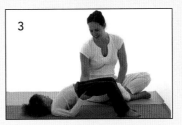
2

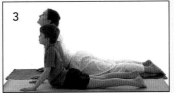
3

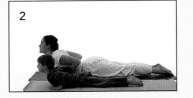
4

14 Cobra pose p.53

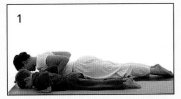
1

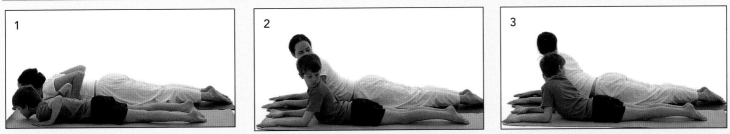
2

3

15 Twisting cobra pose p.54

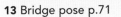

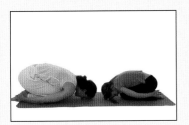

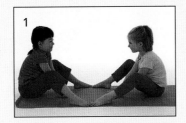
1

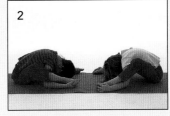
2

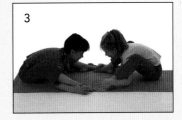
3

16 Child's pose p.74   **17** Tortoise pose p.58

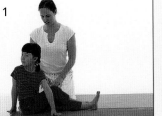
1

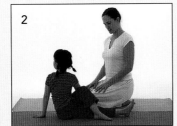
2

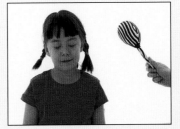

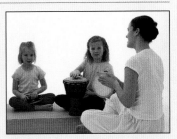

18 Corkscrew pose p.79   **19** Concentration with sound p.114   **20** Chanting p.113

21 Yogic sleep p.115, see 1

Workout for 7–11 year-olds

45 mins

This workout explores the abilities of older children with these dynamic and more complex poses. If children have difficulty with a pose, encourage them to keep trying so that when they accomplish the pose they feel a tremendous sense of achievement.

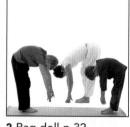
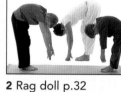
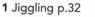

1 Jiggling p.32

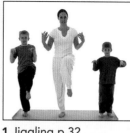

2 Rag doll p.32

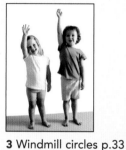

3 Windmill circles p.33

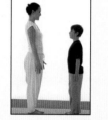

4 Mountain pose p.62

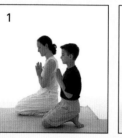

5 Salute to the moon 1 p.85 (or Salute to the moon 2 p.86)

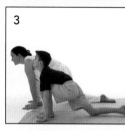
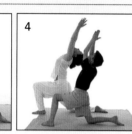
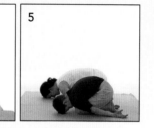
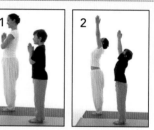

6 Warrior pose p.88

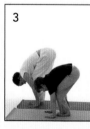
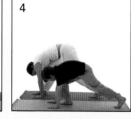
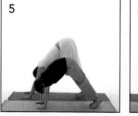
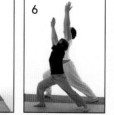
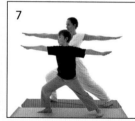

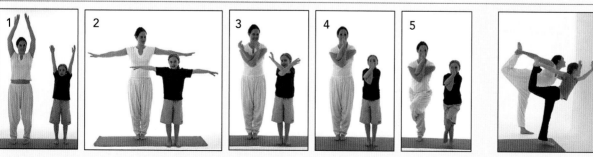

7 Eagle pose p.48

8 King dancer pose p.99

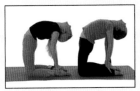 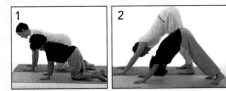

9 Downward dog pose p.44

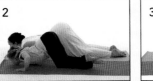 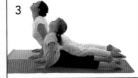 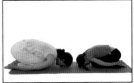

10 Pigeon pose p.49

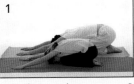 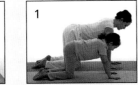 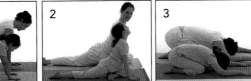

11 Camel pose p.50   **12** Striking cobra pose p.95   **13** Child's pose p.74

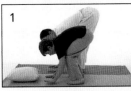 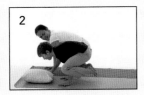 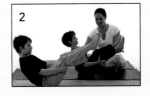 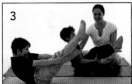

14 Crow pose p.52   **15** Boat pose p.68

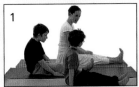 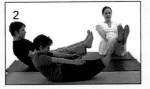 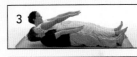 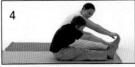

16 Canoe pose p.65   **17** Dynamic sit-up pose p.94

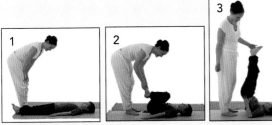 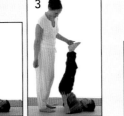 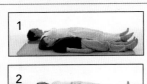 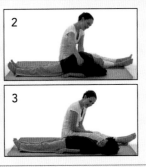

18 Candle pose p.75   **19** Fish pose p.59

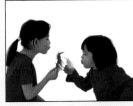 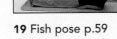 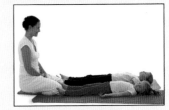

20 Deep breathing p.106   **21** Blowing a fly off the end of the nose p.105   **22** Yogic sleep p.115

Energizing workout

45 mins

These poses invigorate the body and mind. Try to do this workout early in the morning to revitalize you. When a child does a back bend, make sure her tailbone is tucked under and lengthened to protect her lower back.

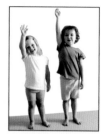

1 Jiggling p.32

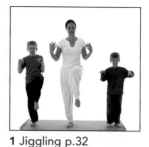

2 Windmill circles p.33

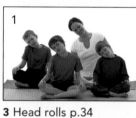 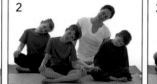 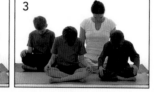

3 Head rolls p.34

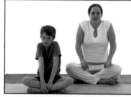

4 Shoulder shrugs p.35

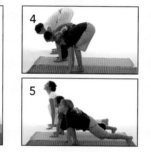 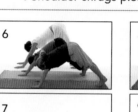 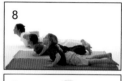 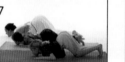 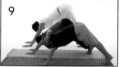

5 Salute to the sun x 3 p.82

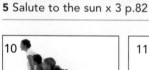 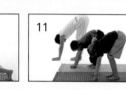 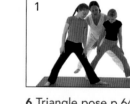 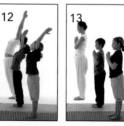 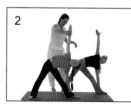

6 Triangle pose p.64

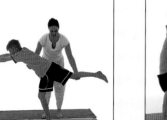 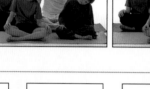 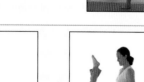 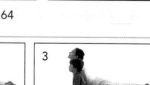

7 Balancing stick pose p.65

8 Upside-down tree pose p.74

9 Cobra pose p.53

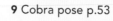

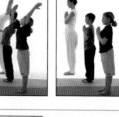

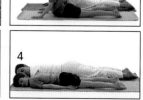

1 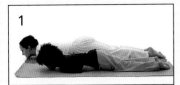 **2** 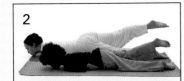 **3** 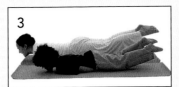 **4**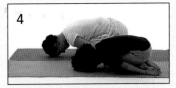

10 Locust pose p.56

1 **2** **3** **4** **5**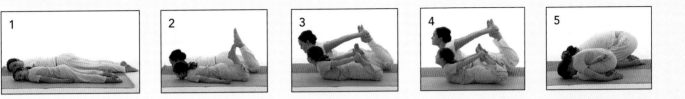

11 Bow pose p.72

1 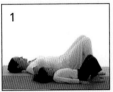 **2** 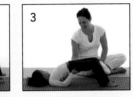 **3** 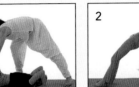 **1** 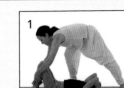 **2** 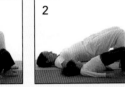 **3**

12 Bridge pose p.71

13 Wheel pose x 3 p.73

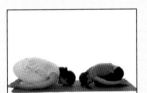 **1** 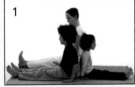 **2** 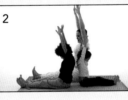 **3**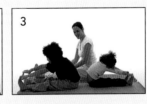

14 Child's pose p.74

15 Jackknife pose p.79

1 **2** **1** **2** **1** **2**

16 Corkscrew pose p.79

17 Rock and roll pose p.92

18 Rolling splits pose p.93

3 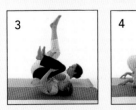 **4** **5** **6**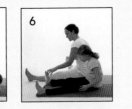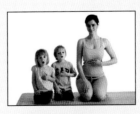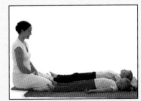

19 Blowing a fly off the
end of the nose p.105

20 Yogic sleep p.115

Calming workout

45 mins

The poses here help to quieten the mind and release tension. Some rest the heart, calming the body, while others encourage contentment and wellbeing. This workout is great for children to do at the end of the day.

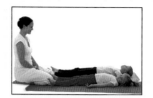

1 Yogic sleep 2–5 minutes p.115
2 Eyes around the clock p.112

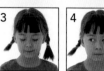

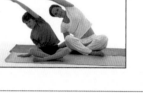 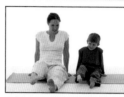 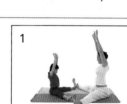

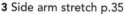 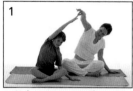

3 Side arm stretch p.35　　**4** Foot rotations p.36　　**5** Leg stretches p.37

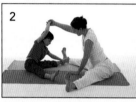 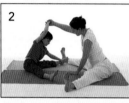 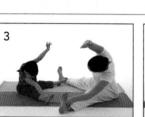 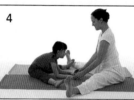 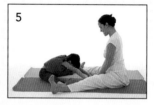

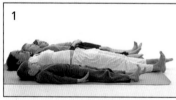

6 Knee to chest p.38

7 Lying side twist p.41

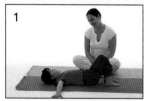 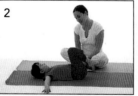 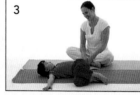 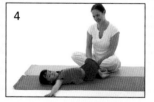

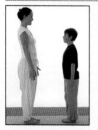 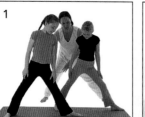 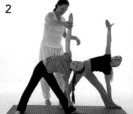 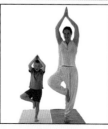
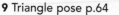

8 Mountain pose p.62　　**9** Triangle pose p.64　　**10** Tree pose p.62

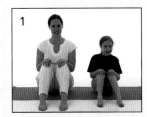 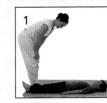 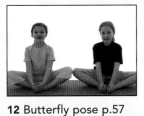 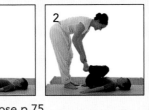 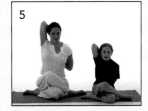

11 Cow face pose p.47

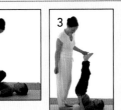 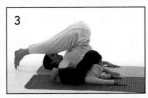

12 Butterfly pose p.57   **13** Candle pose p.75

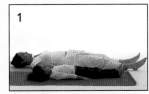 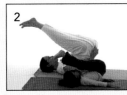

14 Plow pose p.77

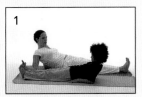 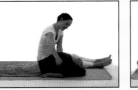 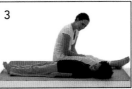

15 Fish pose p.59

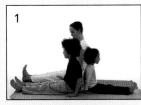 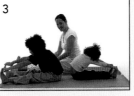 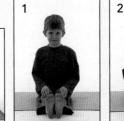

16 Jackknife pose p.79   **17** Lotus pose p.78

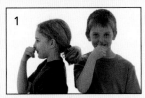 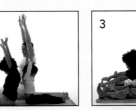 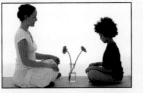 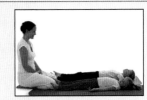

18 Calming breath p.106   **19** Visualization with a flower p.112   **20** Yogic sleep p.115

Index